P9-DOC-206

PRAISE FOR . . .

Strong Women, Strong Bones

"*Strong Women, Strong Bones* provides up-to-date scientific information about osteoporosis, a devastating disease that is preventable and treatable. Comprehensive information on good nutrition, proper exercise, and, when necessary, medication management makes Dr. Nelson's book an excellent resource to help women, and even men, achieve optimal bone health, regardless of their age."
—Sandra C. Raymond, chief executive director,
National Osteoporosis Foundation

"I will strongly recommend this book to all my patients who are concerned about their bones—it is accurate, comprehensive, straightforward, and practical."
—Robert Neer, M.D., director,
Osteoporosis Center, Massachusetts General Hospital

"Nelson and Wernick . . . explain in a clear and friendly manner how bones grow; osteoporosis risk factors; how to adjust the diet to include bone-essential nutrients; the types of . . . exercises that . . . promote maximum bone health; and the latest osteoporosis treatment options. . . . Highly recommended for consumer health collections."
—*Library Journal*

"The authors present the research as it applies to us directly—and in a clear, friendly, accessible style . . . Miriam Nelson and Sarah Wernick are a superb team."
—Fitnesslink.com

"A straightforward, single-purpose guide to [osteoporosis] prevention and treatment . . . Clear, sound help for those at particular risk." —*Kirkus Reviews*

continued on next page . . .

Strong Women Stay Young

"An essential tool for women of all ages." —C. Everett Koop, M.D.,
former United States Surgeon General

"A vitally important book, based on solid scientific research, which for the first time offers hope to the woman who wants to live a long, vigorously active and healthy life to the fullest. It shows clearly that many of the changes associated with aging can be not only delayed, but even reversed."
—Kenneth H. Cooper, M.D., MPH,
author of *The Aerobics Program for Total Well-Being*

"Dr. Nelson has provided women an outstanding opportunity to grow stronger, healthier, and younger." —William J. Evans, Ph.D., director,
Nutrition, Metabolism, and Exercise Laboratory
at the University of Arkansas for Medical Sciences,
and author of *Biomarkers*

"A terrific book! Finally, a science-based program to help women of all ages live strong and vital lives." —Robert N. Butler, M.D., director,
International Longevity Center, Mount Sinai Medical Center

Strong Women Stay Slim

"This book is a gem . . . thoroughly based in science, yet written to help women get started immediately to make their lives better today. It's jam-packed with ready-to-go tools for success." —Barbara Harris, editor in chief,
Shape magazine

"This book is a winner! Miriam Nelson shows women how to take charge and lose weight from a position of strength. Finally there's a weight-loss program that appeals to our intelligence and promotes our fitness."
—Billie Jean King, tennis champion

Most Perigee Books are available at special quantity discounts for bulk purchases for sales promotions, premiums, fund-raising, or educational use. Special books, or book excerpts, can also be created to fit specific needs.

For details, write: Special Markets, The Berkley Publishing Group, 375 Hudson Street, New York, New York 10014.

ALSO BY MIRIAM E. NELSON, PH.D.,
WITH SARAH WERNICK

Strong Women Stay Young
Strong Women Stay Slim
Strong Women, Strong Bones

A PERIGEE BOOK

Strong Women
Eat Well

❖

NUTRITIONAL STRATEGIES
for a
HEALTHY BODY AND MIND

❖

MIRIAM E. NELSON, PH.D.
with
JUDY KNIPE

Every effort has been made to ensure that the information contained in this book is complete and accurate. Neither the publisher nor the author is engaged in rendering professional advice or services to the individual reader. The ideas, procedures, and suggestions contained in the book are not intended as a substitute for consulting with your physician. All matters regarding your health—including possible food allergies and adverse reactions to recipes—require medical supervision. Neither the author nor the publisher shall be liable or responsible for any loss, or damage allegedly arising from any information or suggestion in this book.

A Perigee Book
Published by The Berkley Publishing Group
A division of Penguin Putnam Inc.
375 Hudson Street
New York, New York 10014

The Traditional Healthy Vegetarian Diet Pyramid on page 118 is reprinted with permission of Oldways Preservation & Exchange Trust.

Data for the glycemic index chart on page 47 is reprinted with permission from K. Foster-Powell and J. Brand Miller, "International Tables of Glycemic Index," *American Journal of Clinical Nutrition* 62, no. 4 (October 1995): 871S–890S.

The source for most of the nutrient data listed on pages 89, 90, 105, 106, 129, and 241–249 is Jean A. T. Pennington, Ph.D., R.D., *Bowes and Church's Food Values of Portions Commonly Used*, 17th edition (Lippincott-Raven, 1998). Nutrient data given on page 129 can be found at *www.talksoy.com*.

Copyright © 2001 by Miriam E. Nelson, Ph.D., with Judith B. Knipe
Book design by Deborah Kerner / Dancing Bears Design
Cover design by Michelle Sembler
Cover photo © Millicent Harvey

All rights reserved. This book, or parts thereof,
may not be reproduced in any form without permission.

G. P. Putnam's Sons hardcover edition: July 2001
Perigee trade paperback edition: May 2002

Perigee trade paperback edition ISBN: 0-399-52782-6

Published simultaneously in Canada.

Visit our website at www.penguinputnam.com

The Library of Congress has catalogued the G. P. Putnam's Sons hardcover edition as follows:

Nelson, Miriam E.
Strong women eat well : nutritional strategies for a healthy body and mind /
Miriam E. Nelson with Judy Knipe.
p.   cm.
Includes bibliographical references and index.
ISBN 0-399-14740-3
1. Women—Nutrition. 2. Women—Health and hygiene. I. Knipe, Judy. II. Title.
RA778.N445   2001   00-069677
613.2'082—dc21

Printed in the United States of America

10   9   8   7   6   5   4   3   2

FOR KIN,

WHO NOURISHES MY BODY AND SOUL

Contents

Acknowledgments

◆

Many colleagues, friends, and family members made this book possible. I would like to thank all of them for their valuable guidance and assistance with this book. Doctors Ronenn Roubenoff and Irwin Rosenberg continue to support my writing endeavors—without their support I would not be writing books. Numerous scientists assisted me with various research questions. Special thanks to Doctors William Dietz, Jacob Selhub, Alice Lichtenstein, Christina Economos, Carmen Castaneda, Melissa Bernstein, Kristin Baker, Molly Anderson, and Joel Mason.

Judy Knipe, my collaborator and great friend, has been extraordinary to work with on this book. She is one of the most creative people I know. Not only is she a phenomenal editor but she is a fantastic cook as well. She brought so much to the writing of this book—I enjoyed every minute of working with her.

My research assistant, Rebecca Seguin, worked many evenings and weekends to find relevant research articles and to help me clarify various passages in the book. Her professionalism and good humor were an inspiration throughout the rigorous writing process. She also tested many of the recipes.

My colleagues at Putnam have been incredibly supportive. Stacy Creamer, my editor, has been an ardent champion of Strong Women. Marilyn Ducksworth and Jennifer Swihart in Putnam's publicity department have tirelessly kept the books in the public eye.

Wendy Weil, my dear friend and literary agent, has provided constant support and encouragement throughout my writing career. I would be lost without her.

Michael Sher, Jennifer Layne, MS, CSCS, Kevin Bart, and Cheryl Greene—my colleagues at the Strong Living Company, Inc.—have continued to help me with my overall mission of providing sound, scientific information regarding women's health to the widest possible audience—through *StrongWomen.com* and other media.

Numerous family members and friends assisted me with this book. Tom Earle and Katherine Earle helped to clarify questions I had on organic farming and genetic engineering. Drew Montgomery provided invaluable advice for getting Judy's and my computers to be compatible. Grateful thanks to Rosemarie Garipoli, David Kerr, Ruth Gray, and Robert Bentley, who contributed and tested recipes. Honorable mention to a host of discerning recipe tasters: Lynn Lederer, Rich Meislin, Liz Nelson, Hendrik Uyttendaele, Charles Kaiser, Joe Stouter, John Jesse, Ethel and Paul Hultberg, Susanne Greene, and Tricia Gibney, among others.

Finally, I want to thank my children, Mason, Eliza, and Alexandra.

Preface

————— ❖ —————

I have wanted to write this book for a very long time. For almost two
decades, I have been immersed in the fields of science and public health.
Since 1983, I have been fortunate to work at the Jean Mayer USDA
Human Nutrition Research Center on Aging at Tufts University, where some
of the world's finest research on nutrition and health has been conducted. It
has been enormously exciting to be part of such an undertaking, which has
already made a large contribution to our knowledge and understanding
about this field.

When I first came to Tufts University in 1983, the Center was only a few
years old, but already it was becoming a leader in the field. While my personal research has focused on exercise and women's health, my interest in
nutrition has always remained strong. I have maintained that the key to
health and longevity is a combination of sound nutrition and plenty of
physical activity.

As I wrote this book, friends and family bombarded me with questions
regarding their own nutritional health and the health of their families. Several of these educated women had absorbed and adopted the misconcep-

tions laid out by the media and other sources. They were unsure about their diets and simply wanted to know the truth about nutrition.

I've written this book to bring sound, scientifically based advice to these women as well as thousands of others who care about nutrition. Throughout the book I present many of the findings from recent nutritional studies, information provided so that you will understand the basis for my recommendations. But I urge you not to get bogged down in the minute details of each nutrient. You don't need a doctorate in biochemistry to understand that good nutrition is based on more than just one food. It encompasses the whole diet. My goal with this book is to take the mystery out of nutrition and bring back the pleasure of eating well.

Strong Women Eat Well

❖

CHAPTER 1

Eating Well and Loving It

❖

The science of nutrition is exploding. Almost every day, new research is published showing how what you eat affects your health in specific ways. Good nutrition can promote a sense of well-being in both your body and mind. It can decrease your risk for most of the chronic conditions that we associate with growing older: weight gain, heart disease, high blood pressure, type 2 diabetes, arthritis, osteoporosis, various forms of cancer, and possibly even mental health disorders. And when you combine good nutrition with exercise, you have the most powerful medicine that's available for optimizing your health. A 1993 study of the causes of mortality published in the *Journal of the American Medical Association* estimates that more than 300,000 premature deaths—*deaths that could have been prevented*—occur each year because of poor nutrition and inactivity, a number second only to the 500,000 premature deaths caused each year by cigarette smoking.

The problem is that many nutritional-research findings are reported by the media without context, leading to confusion about the potential benefits and drawbacks of these discoveries. Because our knowledge is expanding so rapidly, and because different studies can produce contradictory results, what we've learned about nutrition in recent years has been obscured by controversy and misconceptions.

The confusion has been fueled by the government and public health community which have, for good reason, adjusted dietary recommendations in response to new research, and by the fad diets popularized by doctors with no training in nutrition. These individuals tend to focus on only one aspect of a food or food group and fail to bring the whole diet into context.

The problem for the public has been compounded by the proliferation of highly processed, convenient, high-calorie, palatable foods that are inexpensive and widely available. These foods are merchandised so aggressively that it is a daunting task to sort out what is healthy from what is not.

An example of where this all leads is the misunderstanding of *fat*. Fat is essential in the human diet. Our bodies need a certain amount of it in order to maintain our skin, immune system, muscles, hormone levels, reproduction, and other important functions. Nutritional research has also shown that several types of fats actually promote health. But by now, dietary fat of any kind has been linked to heart disease and obesity, among other health problems, for so long that a label with the words *fat-free* conveys the misleading subliminal message *This is healthy food.*

Many such foods are more detrimental to health than if they simply contained their original fat content. They have the same amount of calories, and because they are so high in refined sugar, they can cause a high blood glucose response.

EATING WELL TODAY FOR A HEALTHIER TOMORROW

Good nutrition does not come from a pill. The healthiest diet you can eat comes from real foods, whole foods—foods that contain no artificial ingredients, or have not had beneficial substances removed, as refined grains have. Almost all the vitamins, minerals, phytochemicals, and fiber you need, to say nothing of the sheer pleasure of eating, are to be found in food. The best way to get all those nutrients, and get them in the right balance, is to eat a varied diet of whole foods.

It's tempting to think that you can get everything you need to stay healthy by popping a handful of supplements to take the place of the foods you have omitted from your diet, and by taking herbal remedies in pill form that presumably will improve your memory, help prevent colds, or allow you to sleep. Certainly, some supplements have an important role in promoting health, but they are not a substitute for good nutrition because they do not provide the long-term benefits to be had from all the compounds found in food.

Just recently I turned 40. I think of this as an achievement: the stature of early middle age. I'm focused on the here-and-now, on my family, and the way I feel today. But I never lose sight of the way I want to feel thirty or forty years from now, and even beyond that. When I look ahead, I think about my risks for chronic disease, and I know that the best way to grow old with vigor and independence is to pursue the course I'm on now: eating and exercising well, and loving it.

Sometimes it's hard to think about the future until it's there in front of you. But, if eating well can make you feel good right now—can make you look good as well—it will pay off in the future by helping you look and feel your best and by reducing your risk of chronic disease as you grow older.

I care about my health and my state of mind, and I know that most women care about themselves and their families in the same way. But because they are stretched to the limit with work, family, and other commitments, for many women, exercise and eating right are the first to go when time gets tight. In truth, it doesn't take much time to eat well. Knowledge and a little bit of planning can make a huge difference.

WHAT WE EAT IN AMERICA

In Chapter 11, "What's in Food Today?," I talk about the dramatic changes in our food supply that have occurred over the last 50 years. On the plus side of the ledger is the fact that although most of our food is no longer seasonal or locally grown, there are now far more fresh fruits and vegetables available to us year round than ever before. On the minus side, many thousands more processed, unhealthy food products now line our supermarket shelves, and these are the foods many of us choose to eat as a matter of course, as a matter of convenience, and as a matter of subtle persuasion by advertisers.

There have also been profound changes in the way we eat. Fifty years ago we ate family meals together without the television on; we actually ate most of our meals sitting down at a table rather than standing at a counter, at our desks, in the car, or on the run. Most of these changes are for the worse.

Since the 1930s, the U.S. government has been tracking what people eat, information that is important for policy formation, regulations, program planning, and evaluation and education. The National Nutrition Monitoring and Related Research Act of 1990 provides the mandate for large-scale monitoring of Americans' nutrition status and food consumption. I worked aggressively on this bill in 1988 while I was a legislative assistant to Senator Patrick Leahy of Vermont.

Over 16,000 people participate nationwide in the Continuing Survey of Food Intakes by Individuals, popularly known as the "What We Eat in America Survey," which includes more than just what we eat. This is what the most recent data, from 1996, show:

- More than one-half of adults are overweight.
- Forty-four percent of women say they rarely or never exercise vigorously, a number that has been increasing since the 1970s.
- About 57 percent of Americans eat at least one meal away from home on any given day, up from 43 percent in the 1970s. Foods eaten away from home in the mid-1990s accounted for more than 25 percent of total calories and fat intake.
- Women still fail to meet the requirements of several important nutrients: calcium, magnesium, and zinc, and vitamins E and B_6.
- Fruit and vegetable consumption has remained stable over the last couple of decades, with only 55 percent of women even eating fruit or drinking fruit juice on a given day. The average fruit and vegetable consumption for women is 1.5 fruits per day and 3.3 vegetables, far short of what is optimal for good health.
- Grain consumption has risen. Between the late 1970s and the mid-1990s, sales of ready-to-eat cereal increased by 60 percent, and

Americans' consumption of snacks such as crackers, popcorn, pretzels, and corn chips rose by 200 percent.

- Women don't eat enough dietary fiber. On average, women get 14
  grams a day, when they should be eating 20 to 30 grams daily.
- In the 1970s, dietary fat accounted for about 40 percent of the calories in an average American diet. That number has decreased to an
  average of 33 percent. Nevertheless, that percentage is still too high,
  and only one-third of adults consumed 30 percent or less of their
  calories as fat, the figure recommended by nutrition experts (including myself).
- Among children, consumption of milk has decreased by 16 percent
  since the late 1970s, while the consumption of carbonated soft
  drinks has increased by 16 percent. Consumption of noncitrus
  drinks, including grape-, apple-, and other fruit-based mixtures,
  rose by 280 percent.

Among all the changes in the Continuing Survey that have occurred since
the 1970s, four are of special interest and immediate concern. The first
change is a good one: fat consumption has decreased. However, while we
have made great gains in reducing fat intake, it has come with a price. In response to the health recommendation that fat is bad, many in the public now
have a fear of fat. Numerous formerly fat-filled foods have been replaced
by new "fat-free" items, which are chock-full of sugar, salt, additives, and
(often) the same amount of calories as contained in the original foods. People think of these foods as healthy because they are low-fat, so they eat more
of them. But calorie intake has not decreased along with the drop in fat consumption. Another problem is that many of these foods have high amounts
of refined sugar, and they produce a high glycemic response (spiked glucose
and insulin levels in the blood). Over time, eating these foods elevates risk for
heart disease, type 2 diabetes, and obesity.

Second, grain consumption is up significantly. That might be a good
thing if it were whole grains being eaten with such abandon. Unfortunately
we are eating fewer whole grains, such as brown rice and whole-wheat bread,
high-fiber carbohydrates that are digested slowly and satisfy hunger for
longer periods of time. We are, however, consuming more snack foods, white

rice, white pasta, ultra-sweet desserts, and highly processed breakfast cereals than before. These low-fiber, carbohydrate-rich foods are a quick fix for hunger, but because they are quickly digested they satisfy hunger for much shorter periods of time than whole grains. And to the detriment of our health, these foods also produce a high glycemic response.

The third alarming trend is the increasingly sedentary lifestyle of Americans, which has so many deleterious consequences for our health. Finally, the fourth change is the growing epidemic of obesity in America, which *is* the consequence of the first three trends. The epidemic is not just among adults but, even more worrisome, among our children.

Food supply gone awry

In the early 1950s, there were about 2,000 different food items on sale at the local grocery store. By the 1980s, that number had grown to 5,000 items, and today more than 40,000 different foods are being sold at the average supermarket, with about 60,000 or more in a superstore. Thirteen thousand new food products are introduced each year.

Few new varieties of apples or brown rice are being grown and marketed. The boom is in prepared meals, processed foods, sodas, snack bars, refined breakfast cereals, and other unwholesome foods. The good news is that because many more consumers are aware of good nutrition, they are demanding healthier food products. In response, some food manufacturers are developing and marketing healthier choices.

Shopping for food at a supermarket has become much more difficult. I admit that I have a certain nostalgia for the local grocery of my childhood. My mother and I knew the owner—he even bought a puppy from us. The store was about the size of most people's garages, with many fewer choices than there are today, and we could easily figure out which fresh foods we wanted for our meals. Now when I go to the supermarket with my children, it takes forever, and it's difficult navigating through the multitude of processed foods to find the few whole-food items that I need. In fact, there are so many products, so many labels to read, so many health factors to consider, that sometimes it's hard to grasp just how unhealthy a seemingly reasonable, time-saving choice may actually be.

The relentless merchandising of food products has changed the way we eat. Don't get me wrong. I love the fact that I can now buy freshly squeezed orange juice and kiwis as well as a variety of whole-grain cereals at the supermarket. It's just that these few amenities are overshadowed by a super-abundance of tempting processed foods that do not promote health.

Restaurant meals: where's the real "value"?

"What We Eat in America," the survey described previously, shows that well over half of us eat at least one meal away from home on any given day. One third of those meals are from fast-food restaurants. Although fast food is notorious for being, on average, higher in fat—especially saturated fat—and lower in fiber and fruits and vegetables than home-cooked food, the same is true of almost any meal you eat in a restaurant.

It's not surprising that there is a strong relationship between frequency of eating in restaurants and obesity. It's not just because the food is higher in fat than it would be if you prepared it at home, it is because the portions are obscenely large. Fast-food restaurants are not the only offenders; other family restaurants and even more expensive ones are serving just as much, that is, far too much, food. My husband and I are big eaters, but most of the time we can't come close to finishing a full meal at a restaurant.

Americans expect to get "value" for their money: the larger the portion, the greater the value. That's why restaurants are serving such large meals to an increasingly obese public that is always eager for more. This trend is unfortunate; eating larger quantities of nutritionally deficient food is not the way to go. In other countries, especially in Europe, value in a meal comes from the taste and quality of the meal, not from the quantity of food piled on a plate.

One of the best means of restaurant portion control that I know of, and one that my family and I practice, is simply to ask the waiter to split the meal in two. The cook usually will do this for a minimal charge, and you get just as many vegetables but only half the (huge) portion of the meat, fish, or main part of the entrée. That way, we don't overeat, and we have spent less too, getting real "value" for our money. Other people I know simply ask for doggie bags instead of eating everything on their plates.

Of course, it's not just restaurants that offer such "value." I'm sure the first mountain of mashed potatoes many of us ever saw was not dished up by the local Hi-Cal Diner: It was served at home. Start early with your kids. At home, you can serve large portions of fresh vegetables and fruits and adequate and satisfying portions of protein-rich foods and starches. That way, you'll help shape their concept of the type and amount of food they need in order to feel full. It's the first step on the road to healthy eating and long-term weight control.

EATING WELL AND LOVING IT

A *good* meal—as opposed to a *huge* meal—is one of life's greatest pleasures. It does far more than appease hunger and provide the benefits of nutrition. For me, much of the pleasure in eating comes from sharing the time with my family, or if I am away, with colleagues and friends.

The lost art of pleasurable eating

We are so fortunate to live in a time of plenty and in an era of scientific discovery. And though we should be enjoying the benefits of recent studies that show the strong link between good health and good nutrition, many of us have lost touch with real, wholesome food and the pleasures of mealtime.

We all know the reasons why: work schedules that extend into the evening hours (both in one- and two-parent households); children's after-school activities, many of which involve parents as well; television, which hinders almost any continuous conversation; the seductions of computer games and the Web. With all this competition, there's scarcely any time left for meals that are enjoyed for themselves, whether eaten alone or shared with others. I think this is one of the worst changes in the way we live, and it has had a harmful effect on our nutrition and health.

At home, I look forward to evening meals, when my family sits down around the dinner table, sometimes with neighbors and visiting friends, and we catch up on the events of our day and share good conversation and delicious food. It's true that this rosy picture is not realized every night. There are times when my husband or I are away from home and times when one or all of the children are eating elsewhere. But the habit, or ritual if you like, of sitting down together without the television on has been established. That time together makes a difference to all of us.

Fads, food obsessions, and extreme eating

From aphrodisiacs to cold remedies, there have always been fads and obsessions about food. Some are based on actual science, usually one small piece of information isolated from a larger body of science; some are based on quasi-science—the blanket condemnation of fat is a good example—and some are simply *bubbameisses,* tales your grandmother told you.

Three areas of nutrition currently preoccupy many Americans: fats (all bad), proteins (eat all you can for rapid weight loss), and carbohydrates (they're fattening; avoid them). These are extreme positions, and they are held by those who have the most to gain: the biased scientists who sell the fad diets, and the food industry that creates, promotes, and sells the processed foods that support the diets. The facts, as opposed to the fads, are that each of these foods is essential to our health if eaten in the amounts that are recommended.

Such phobias and obsessions not only harm our health, they prevent us from enjoying food. I can't tell you how often I've been out for a meal with the kind of person who is so ruled by fear of fat or carbohydrates that she is almost paralyzed by the act of ordering food—so what she has is just a salad with dressing on the side. Her usual lunch is a bag of fat-free pretzels, a container of fat-free yogurt (sometimes it's sugar-free, too—I can't imagine what's in it), and a diet soda, which she eats at her desk. Where is the pleasure? Where is the nutritional boost she needs to sustain her for the rest of the afternoon?

One of the themes of this book is that we need to be aware of what we eat. Awareness is not vigilance, and the fear of food can be as unhealthy and as reckless as indifference to it.

I am very fortunate that my work has given me the opportunity to meet and speak with women all over America, and in other countries as well. Most women tell me they know that good nutrition is the key to good health, but they are not always sure what their nutritional goals should be and how to achieve them.

I believe that taking care of your body is part of your human job description, and the best way to start is by eating well. I wrote *Strong Women Eat Well* to help you create your own healthy and pleasurable way to eat, one that will optimize your nutritional status and, at the same time, reflect your food preferences and your lifestyle. For me, good nutrition and pleasure are concepts that embrace the entire world of food. I strongly believe that the more variety of fresh whole foods you eat, coupled with regular exercise, the healthier you will be.

Here's to your health!

CHAPTER 2

The New National Guidelines

A Solid Base
for Optimal Nutrition

❖

The nutritional recommendations I make in this book are based on several guidelines published and promoted by the national government: the Food Guide Pyramid (FGP), the Dietary Guidelines for Americans, the Recommended Daily Allowances (RDAs), and the Dietary Reference Intakes (DRIs). The FGP focuses on foods, while the Dietary Guidelines outline broader aspects of fitness, nutrition, and health. The RDAs and the DRIs focus on specific nutrients.

Recent changes in government nutrition guidelines have caused some confusion in the public, due more to revised terminology than to doubts about the guidelines' merit as the basis for creating a nutritional plan. For instance, RDAs seem to have morphed into DRIs. In fact, these are two distinctly separate entities, but in the mind of the consumer, they have been melded into a single set of values. The particulars of the RDAs and DRIs are discussed at the back of this book.

The validity of the FGP and the Dietary Guidelines is undoubted. Both are formulated from the findings of thousands of laboratory and epidemiological studies and the recommendations of hundreds of scientists and other nutrition professionals. The guidelines serve as an excellent base for good health, but I believe that they can and should be adapted to each individual's needs in order to optimize nutritional status. As an example, later in the book I recommend that you eat the lowest number of grain servings (and at least half of them should be whole grains) and the highest number of fruits and vegetables suggested in the FGP. Both recommendations fall well within the government guidelines.

THE FOOD GUIDE PYRAMID

In the early 1990s, the Food Guide Pyramid, subtitled "A Guide to Daily Food Choices," was developed by the departments of Health and Human Services (HHS) and Agriculture (USDA). The pyramid is based on food groups such as fruits and grains instead of on nutrients such as specific vitamins and minerals. It illustrates in a clear, graphic way how many servings from each food group we need to eat every day in order to be healthy.

The pyramid was an important step in nutrition guidelines. First, its focus is the whole diet: it includes the full range of food groups, not just one component of what we eat. Second, because *all* foods fit into the pyramid, whatever your food preferences, religious beliefs, or heritage, you can use it as the basis for your own diet.

How many servings should I eat?

The shape of the pyramid itself and the recommended number of servings per day for each group are useful tools to help you create a diet with the right amount of calories to maintain a healthy weight. The five bottom food groups within the three lower levels are packed with nutrient-rich foods. The tip of the pyramid shows the food groups that should be consumed in moderation for optimal health and weight control—Fats, Oils & Sweets.

If you eat the lower number of recommended servings in each food group, you will consume about 1,600 calories a day, the amount necessary for many sedentary women and most older adults. If you eat from the middle range, you'll consume about 2,200 calories, the amount necessary for

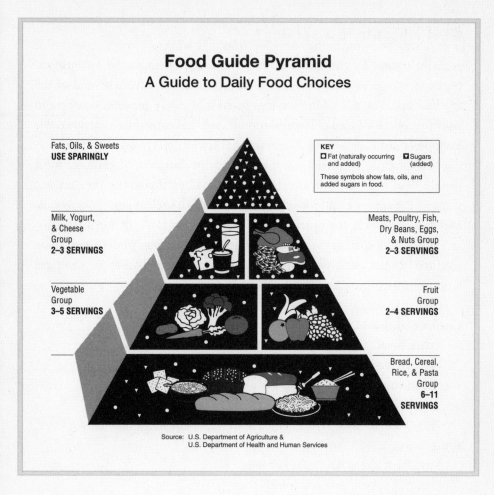

Food Guide Pyramid
A Guide to Daily Food Choices

Fats, Oils, & Sweets
USE SPARINGLY

KEY
◻ Fat (naturally occurring   ◼ Sugars
  and added)   (added)

These symbols show fats, oils, and
added sugars in food.

Milk, Yogurt,
& Cheese
Group
2–3 SERVINGS

Meats, Poultry, Fish,
Dry Beans, Eggs,
& Nuts Group
2–3 SERVINGS

Vegetable
Group
3–5 SERVINGS

Fruit
Group
2–4 SERVINGS

Bread, Cereal,
Rice, & Pasta
Group
**6–11
SERVINGS**

Source: U.S. Department of Agriculture &
           U.S. Department of Health and Human Services

most teenage girls, active women, and many sedentary men. The upper range provides about 2,800 calories, the amount necessary for most teenage boys, active men, and very active women. This represents a wide range of energy intakes—1,600 to 2,800 calories—that is appropriate for most Americans, although it doesn't necessarily meet the needs of every individual, such as elite athletes who must eat in excess of 4,000 or 5,000 calories a day to maintain ideal body weight.

What amounts to a serving?

A major reason for the rise in obesity in America is that we eat enormous portions of everything, from snacks to full meals, and from several of the food groups. The size of the servings listed in the FGP may not conform to your preconceived idea of the amount of food that constitutes a serving. For example, most bagels that you buy in a bakery or deli are actually four serving sizes of grain, or about half the entire daily allotment of grain for most people. Take a careful look at the FGP portion sizes. If possible, measure out some of the amounts of foods that you usually eat, such as pasta, rice, meats, and dairy products, then measure out the same foods in portion sizes listed in the FGP. Comparing the actual quantities will help you understand where you need to cut back, where you need to increase, and what are the right amounts for you.

Grains, cereal, and pasta
  1 slice bread
  1 ounce ready-to-eat cereal
  ½ cup cooked cereal, rice, or pasta
  ¼ large bagel

Fruit
  1 medium apple, banana, or orange
  ½ cup chopped (raw or cooked) fruit
  ½ cup fruit juice

Vegetable
  1 cup raw leafy vegetable (lettuce, spinach, etc.)
  ½ cup other vegetables, cooked or chopped raw
  ½ cup vegetable juice

Milk, yogurt, and cheese
  1 cup milk or yogurt
  1½ ounces hard cheese
  2 ounces processed cheese

Meat, poultry, fish, eggs, dried beans, and nuts
   2 to 3 ounces cooked lean meat, fish, or poultry
   ½ cup cook dried beans
   1 egg, 2 tablespoons peanut butter, and ½ cup nuts all equal
      1 ounce meat

Some people reject the pyramid because of its simplicity, but as a scientist interested in public health I *welcome* the simplicity. Anyone can look at it and ask, "Did I get the right number of servings in each category? Did I get three to five servings of vegetables, did I get two to four servings of fruits?" If you are like most American women, you didn't.

The choice is yours

I will be the first to say that it is possible to eat very poorly following the FGP, just as it is possible to eat very well. For instance, if you choose to eat all of your vegetables from cans; if you choose to eat your fruits in the form of sugar-rich desserts; if you choose to eat fatty meats that are processed with large amounts of salt, sugar, and nitrates; if the only grains you eat are highly refined—no matter how many or how few servings you eat, you will not be eating well.

And the reverse is true. If you choose to eat fresh fruits and vegetables, whole grains such as brown rice and whole wheat bread, lean meats, cold-water fish, and sensible amounts of dairy foods, fats, and sugars, you will be eating very well indeed!

Adapting the FGP for your own food preferences

By now, twelve alternative FGPs have been published, each with a different ethnic, medical, or population perspective (see Resources for a listing).

At Tufts University, colleagues developed the Food Guide Pyramid for People over 70 Years of Age, which provides extra advice for older adults to help them meet their unique nutritional needs, including more guidance on getting enough fluids and some supplements. There is a pyramid for the very popular and healthy Mediterranean Diet, which focuses on the typical dietary patterns of Mediterranean cultures. There is a Vegetarian Diet Pyramid (which you will find in Chapter 8), and pyramids for children and for Asian, Catalan, Latin American, and other diets.

Each of these FGPs has amended the food groups to conform to the particular dietary needs or food preferences of the group concerned. For example, while there is still a meat group in the Mediterranean Diet, it has been minimized, and a fish group has been added. The diet plans from all of these pyramids are sound and healthy, but each one has been tailored to the specific foods that are ordinarily grown and consumed in those regions and cultures. These food pyramids are developed by a number of different organizations ranging from universities to special interest groups, and I believe that for the most part, the pyramids are sound and helpful.

Dietary Guidelines for Americans

In May 2000, the USDA and HHS released the fifth *Dietary Guidelines for Americans*. Federal dietary guidelines, or goals, developed by the USDA and HHS were first published in 1977 and since then have undergone five revisions. I began working in the field of nutrition in the early 1980s, and I've seen most of the revisions. In my opinion, each set gets better and better, with the fifth edition the best by far.

The reason for this high rating is the first guideline, "Aim for Fitness," which highlights the importance of physical activity and weight control as nutritional issues for optimal health. With over half of the population sedentary and overweight, this is a critical guideline. Finally, after twenty-three years, policy makers realize that nutrition and physical activity go hand in hand. And, as you will see, these guidelines encourage you to use the FGP as your guide to selecting healthy foods.

These two guidelines form the basis of federal food, nutrition education, and information programs. As you can see, they have been expanded to include not only guidance on nutrition, but on other lifestyle factors as well, especially fitness and weight control for overall health. (See the Resources section for information about obtaining the entire Dietary Guidelines

DIETARY GUIDELINES FOR AMERICANS

AIM FOR FITNESS...

▲ Aim for a healthy weight.

▲ Be physically active each day.

BUILD A HEALTHY BASE...

■ Let the Pyramid guide your food choices.

■ Choose a variety of grains daily, especially whole grains.

■ Choose a variety of fruits and vegetables daily.

■ Keep food safe to eat.

CHOOSE SENSIBLY...

● Choose a diet that is low in saturated fat and cholesterol and moderate in total fat.

● Choose beverages and foods to moderate your intake of sugars.

● Choose and prepare foods with less salt.

● If you drink alcoholic beverages, do so in moderation.

...for good health

booklet.) No doubt, in the next few years additional and/or updated guidelines on nutrition will be issued by the government based on new research.

I hope that you will use these guidelines and the information and recommendations that are the heart of this book to create your own individual nutrition and fitness programs.

CHAPTER 3

Water

Our Most Essential Nutrient

❖

We tend to take water for granted, and yet our lives depend on it. Water is our most important nutrient, second only to oxygen in providing what our bodies need to survive. It is the basic medium in which all life-sustaining biochemical processes occur.

Water, in any one of dozens of chemical formulations, makes up by far the largest part of human body weight: about 55 percent for a woman and about 65 percent for a man. Imagine the human body as a ripe plum, and then think about its dried counterpart, the prune. You will then be able to appreciate how a lack of water could impair the way the body works—not to mention how it looks. When I don't get enough water, especially in the summer, I start to feel like a prune.

WATER'S VITAL ROLES IN THE BODY

As water enters, moves through, and exits the body, it is transformed into dozens of fluids that perform a multitude of critically important functions. Here are a few of the ways water works in the body.

Catalyst for digestion and absorption

During digestion the food you eat undergoes a process known as metabolism, in which vital nutrients are absorbed and utilized by the body. Saliva, whose main component is water, assists in the process by lubricating the throat and helping to carry food to the stomach. Gastric juices in the stomach and intestine provide further assistance in helping to break down the food, making it possible to absorb nutrients in the gut.

Expressway for nutrients and waste

Blood, also composed primarily of water, works with the lymphatic system as the body's internal highway for transporting nutrients, hormones, and waste from one site to another. Nutrients, such as glucose, fatty acids, and amino acids, are delivered to muscles; and hormones, such as estrogen, are transported to bones, brain, and other tissues that need them.

Water is utilized in the disposal of carbon dioxide and other metabolic waste via blood plasma, while urine and stool (a large percentage of which is water) carry waste products that are eliminated from the body.

Regulator of body temperature

Sweating is one way the body regulates its internal temperature, particularly during heavy exercise. When your internal temperature is elevated, the capillaries open up, blood flows toward the skin, and the skin perspires. The skin is cooled by evaporation, cooling the blood in the capillaries close to the skin, which in turn travels back to help cool deeper body chambers.

Universal lubricant

Without water you would be like the Tin Man in *The Wizard of Oz*. Where he used oil, you use fluids. For instance, the water sacs between joints—also known as bursas—act as cushions and lubricants to facilitate comfortable movement. Water also keeps your tongue and eyes moist, and it's the main

If you're older . . .

Older women need the same amount of water every day as younger women. But because their thirst centers are less acute than when they were younger, they must learn to drink *more than their body tells them* they need. By the time they actually begin to feel thirsty, mild dehydration has begun, and they are, in a sense, running on empty.

Older women should drink 8 glasses of fluid spaced at intervals throughout the day, even if they don't feel the thirst.

component of the cerebrospinal fluid that protects the brain and spinal cord and the amniotic fluid that surrounds a fetus.

Regulator of blood pressure

The volume of blood plasma is a major determinant of blood pressure and cardiovascular function. In the case of dehydration, blood volume is decreased and blood pressure can become dangerously low.

Conversely, excess water retention—sometimes the case with specific types of heart disease—increases blood volume, which can put extra pressure on the arteries and cause high blood pressure.

HOW THE BODY MAINTAINS WATER BALANCE

Two of the body's major organs—the brain and the kidneys—are largely responsible for maintaining an exquisite balance of fluid in your body.

The brain

The amount of water you drink is influenced by thirst and satiety, sensations that are recognized by your mouth, brain, and nerves. Thirst and satiety are such complex bodily functions that they are not yet fully comprehended by the scientific community.

What we do know is that when you take in too little water, your blood becomes too concentrated, your mouth becomes dry, and your brain signals thirst, so you start to drink. But very often, there is a lag time, and the degree of thirst that you feel does not always accurately reflect the extent of your dehydration.

Children, whose thirst centers are more acute, respond to dehydration quickly, in the most direct and spontaneous way. They are constantly thirsty, always drinking fluids, and, unless they are ill, manage to keep themselves well hydrated.

However, as you age, your thirst centers become less acute, the signals they send are dulled and do not respond as well to dehydration, and you are not as likely to drink as much as you need.

The ins and outs of fluid balance

Daily fluid intake for a typical sedentary person
8 cups from drinks, soups
4 cups from foods
1 cup produced in the body from metabolism

Daily loss of fluid for a typical person
8 cups in urine
½ cup fluid in stools
½ cup fluid in sweat
4 cups fluid in insensible water loss from skin and respiration

If you are a very active person, these numbers change dramatically: Increase the amounts for intake and loss, especially loss of fluids in urine and sweat.

When you drink too much water, your stomach becomes stretched and signals your brain to stop drinking.

The kidneys

The kidneys have a strong regulatory effect on blood pressure. When the amount of water in your body increases, so does your blood pressure, and, conversely, when you have too little water in your body, your blood pressure goes down. The kidneys, using very specialized cells designed for that purpose, can sense blood pressure.

When the bloodstream carries chemical waste and water to your kidneys, it is the kidneys' job to filter the blood and remove harmful waste products.

When your blood is at very high volume, your kidneys sense that the blood is too dilute. In order to help bring the balance of compounds in the blood back to normal, the kidneys filter the water out of the bloodstream into urine.

If your blood is too viscous because you are dehydrated, the kidneys do everything they can to conserve fluid in order to keep blood at the proper concentrate.

How does your body get water?

You get 60 to 70 percent of your water from drinking liquids. The best sources are water, juice, and milk. Caffeinated drinks such as soda, coffee, and tea have a diuretic effect, causing them to lose about 30 to 50 percent of their water. Even so, they are still sources of fluid.

Most of your remaining fluid intake comes from water that is part of solid food. Ideal sources are fruits, vegetables, especially lettuce and other leafy greens, and liquid or semiliquid foods such as soups. But even such unlikely foods as chicken breast (about 65 percent water), cheese (cheddar is 30 percent water), and biscuits (25 percent water) are respectable sources of water.

About 5 percent of the water your body uses is generated within the body itself through metabolic processes.

Each and every day the body performs the remarkable feat of keeping itself in fluid balance. What makes this more amazing is that even though the human body is 60 percent water, you rarely have imbalances of more than a cup of fluid. Your weight, measured day to day, is more or less constant, with minor fluctuations during the premenstrual cycle. Water balance is critical in order for the brain to function, muscles to contract, and blood to flow. It is the body's response to its own need for the water that is necessary for all of your bodily functions.

HOW MUCH DO YOU NEED?

It is an unfortunate truth that some people do not drink as much fluid as they need to get the maximum health benefits. Obviously, most of us take in "enough" fluid to get by, but we do not take in an amount that is optimal. The information that follows will help you establish your own guidelines for how much fluid you should drink every day to optimize your health.

Women

Generally, your water needs depend on how much energy you expend. For most women to maintain body temperature and water balance, the rule of

What is a fluid cup?

A fluid cup measures 8 fluid ounces. In terms of your need for fluids, however, some drinks are more equal than others. Water and juice are the most beneficial fluids to drink, followed by low-fat milk. Carbonated sodas are also a source of fluids. An 8-ounce glass of any of these beverages counts for a full 8 ounces of your daily fluid intake. But, because they increase urine production and fluid loss, caffeinated and alcoholic beverages count for only half their measurable amounts: each 8-ounce cup of them you drink counts for only ½ cup, or 4 ounces, of fluid.

thumb is you should drink eight 8-ounce cups, increasing that a
additional one cup for each half hour of moderate exercise y
the day.

Illness

You will need extra fluids when you are sick.

- Vomiting or diarrhea drain your body of fluids and salt.
- Fever causes extra water and electrolyte loss through perspiration.
- People suffering from certain chronic diseases, such as diabetes,
  need extra water.
- Any disruption in the body's normal functioning, such as shock or
  emotional stress, can cause mild dehydration.

Certain prescription medications—diuretics, some antibiotics, and antigout
drugs—may interact with water and electrolytes to cause an imbalance,
which makes proper hydration all the more critical.

Lactation

Nursing mothers need to be especially diligent about drinking extra water. In
fact, nursing mothers need to drink at least 16 cups of fluid every day, or
double the normal amount, depending on the size of the baby and whether
the child is getting any other supplemental drink or food.

Mild dehydration during lactation will not cut down on your milk production, but it will make you tired. Moderate dehydration can deplete your
milk production and make you even more tired. Fortunately, most nursing
mothers have a very good thirst and drink plenty of fluids.

Exercise

Excessive water and electrolyte loss during exercise is primarily a result of an
increased amount of sweat generated because working muscles are creating
heat. During strenuous exertion, so much body water is lost-—6 to 10 percent

Electrolytes—maintaining a balance

Electrolytes are salts, or mineral compounds, that dissolve in water and break up into particles that can have positive or negative charges. Electrolytes—namely potassium, sodium, and chloride—are needed to maintain the proper balance of fluids inside and outside your cells (two-thirds of body fluids are inside cells and one third of fluids are outside of cells). Under normal circumstances, fluid balance in the body is a given, but when you experience excessive sweating, vomiting, or diarrhea, your electrolyte balance may become upset and you can become very ill. The best way to restore this balance is to drink plenty of fluids (sports drinks can help) and eat as you normally would.

How a sports drink can help

If you are exercising strenuously, even indoors, for longer than two to three hours, or if you are exercising outdoors in the heat for any length of time, an electrolyte-enhanced sports drink is appropriate. When choosing such a drink, keep these tips in mind:

- *Water* is the most important component.
- *Glucose polymers,* which are more easily absorbed by the small intestine and cause less gastric distress than plain sugar, should make up no more than 7 percent of the sports drink. (More than 10 percent glucose concentration can cause cramps and diarrhea, so be sure to check the sports drink label carefully.)
- *Electrolytes,* such as sodium, are constituents in most sports drinks because they help replenish the electrolytes lost in sweat as well as helping your small intestine absorb the water from the drink.

Keep in mind that the sports drink industry is a $1 billion market. Some people enjoy the taste of sports drinks for hydration, but unless

you are working out at high intensities for long durati‍
drinks are unnecessary. There is one other use for sports drinks.
cause the electrolytes and glucose polymers in these drinks are easily
absorbed, they are sometimes recommended by doctors to replenish
body fluids if you have had diarrhea or vomiting.

can be lost during a marathon—that very often the kidneys stop urine out-
put to offset the loss from sweat.

Here is a guide for determining when to drink fluids and what fluids to
drink when exercising:

Short-duration exercise (less than 1 hour)
Stay hydrated by drinking water or any other dilute beverage 30 minutes before you begin to exercise. Unless you are exercising at a high intensity, you
won't need special drinks or a special hydration schedule—just keep well hydrated with water or juices after exercise.

Medium-duration exercise (1 to 3 hours)
Drink 1 to 2 cups of water within the hour before the event. During the
event, drink ½ to 1 cup of fluids every 15 minutes. Depending on the intensity of exercise, drink either water or dilute carbohydrate sports drinks.

Long-duration events (over 3 hours)
Follow the advice for medium-duration events, but during the exercise drink
dilute carbohydrate electrolyte sports drinks to maintain your body's blood
glucose and electrolyte levels.

Recovery
Whatever the length of your event, it is important for you to replenish fluids
after exercise. Drink plenty of water, fruit juices, or other beverages within the
hour after your event. In long-duration events, it is important to weigh yourself
before and after the event. By an hour or two after the event, you should be sufficiently rehydrated so that you are within a few pounds of your prerace weight.

Don't let incontinence slow you down

Many women, especially women who have just had a baby or those who are older, tell me that they reduce or limit their intake of fluids because of incontinence.

The three major kinds of incontinence are:

Stress incontinence

The muscles on your pelvic floor support the uterus and bladder and control voluntary urination. These muscles can be weakened or damaged because of pregnancy or childbirth, especially multiple childbirths, or from estrogen loss. Stress incontinence occurs when abdominal pressure—from a cough, a laugh, a body movement, or a sneeze—causes a sudden increase in pressure on your bladder wall and bladder sphincter, triggering a urine leak.

Urge incontinence

Urinary tract infection (UTI), or inflammation of the bladder, causes the bladder muscles to spasm, or contract uncontrollably, prompting urine leakage. It is possible for you to have both stress and urge incontinence simultaneously.

Overflow incontinence

Although you may feel no urge to urinate, your bladder fills to capacity and excess urine spills out. This condition is most common in diabetics, but also occurs in women who "hold it" for too long (five to six hours at a time) over the course of years. Stroke, spinal cord injuries, multiple sclerosis, and other neurological disorders can cause overflow incontinence in women and men. Enlarged prostate in men is a frequent cause of urine overflow.

What can help

If incontinence becomes persistent, consult your doctor. There are sound and successful treatments for the condition, which include medications to improve urethral muscle tone, surgery to return the bladder to its original location, and pelvic muscle exercises (Kegel exercises, see below).

A study from the University of Alabama has shown that older women suffering from urge incontinence can benefit most from a combination of drug treatments and behavioral therapy, or biofeedback, as well as the Kegel exercises. Your doctor should be able to discuss with you the best options for your particular situation.

Changes in your diet can also make a difference. Try to eliminate, or at least limit your intake of, caffeinated and carbonated beverages—coffee, tea, soda—artificial sweeteners, chocolate, tomatoes, and hot spices, all of which can aggravate incontinence.

Among the lifestyle changes you can make are to stop smoking; take precautions to assure that you are not constipated, which can exacerbate incontinence; maintain your proper weight; avoid alcohol; and do Kegel exercises.

Kegel exercises

These exercises, developed by Dr. Arnold Kegel, can help strengthen the muscles of your pelvic floor. The technique, which involves squeezing and tightening those muscles, is best taught to you by your healthcare provider during a vaginal exam. She will be able help you locate the muscles and describe how you should feel as you are doing the exercises. See the Resources section for more information.

Climate and altitude

Climate has an important effect in increasing the body's water requirements. Depending on how hot it is, your need for fluids can double in warm weather even though your thirst center may lag behind. Be sure that you have ready access to a source of water during hot weather, and drink often. In addition, when you are at high altitudes, you will lose water or become dehydrated faster than you would at or near sea level.

Don't restrict your fluid intake

When you reduce your consumption of liquids, your urine becomes more concentrated, which in turn causes your bladder to contract in order to rid itself of that concentrated urine as quickly as possible. Limiting intake can also cause constipation, urinary tract infections (UTIs), dehydration, and kidney stones, all of which can increase incontinence. Continue to drink as much water as your body needs to maintain all its vital functions, and urinate as soon as you feel the urge, or every three to four hours, whichever comes first.

DEHYDRATION IS DANGEROUS TO YOUR HEALTH

The early stages of dehydration, or deprivation of fluids, may not seem alarming. But unremedied, progressive dehydration is extremely dangerous, and its debilitating effects can escalate rapidly due to loss of the electrolytes that help regulate so many of your vital functions.

If you detect any of the early signs of dehydration in yourself or someone else, immediate intake of fluids is the only answer. Later signs require the attention of a doctor. This is what to watch for:

- Mild dehydration (1 to 2 percent): thirst, fatigue, weakness, vague discomfort, loss of appetite
- Moderate dehydration (3 to 6 percent): nausea, flushed skin, severe fatigue, tingling hands and feet, headaches, increased body temperature, increased respiration and pulse, impatience, apathy, dry mouth, difficulty concentrating, headache, sleepiness
- Severe dehydration (7 to 10 percent): swelled tongue, beginning of kidney failure, dizziness, muscle spasms, loss of balance, delirium, collapse, exhaustion, death

Unhealthy dieting can cause dehydration

There are several kinds of weight loss diets that can cause danger-ous dehydration. Those most at risk are:

Women with eating disorders who purge themselves with enemas or induce vomiting lose fluid by doing so and also lose important electrolytes and other nutrients. This combination puts them at increased risk for serious dehydration, not to mention other life-threatening complications.

Women who eat a high-protein diet are on a much more subtle but equally dangerous path, and they put themselves at special risk for dehydration. You may seem to be losing weight quickly, but in fact al-most all of the loss is water. When you lose water from your body, you are losing an important element of your body. Water is the easiest, fastest constituent of your body to lose, and along with water loss, you will deplete your body of protein from your muscles and calcium from your bones.

People who exercise in the heat wearing a lot of clothing or wet suits as a means of weight control are also in serious danger. This oc-curs most often among wrestlers and other athletes who need to meet restricted weight categories for their sport. Every year, people (usu-ally young adults) die from the practice, which generates a superabun-dance of sweat and results in severe dehydration and kidney failure.

I strongly urge you to avoid any of these practices, as they are ex-tremely dangerous and can even be deadly.

STRONG STRATEGIES FOR OPTIMAL HYDRATION

I am one of those people who have a hard time getting enough fluid every day. I forget to drink. Many days I'll get to the end of the workday, and I'll realize that all I had to drink was a cup of hot tea at 6 a.m. and a little juice at lunch. It's no wonder I'm so tired. Over the past couple of years, this has been one of the dietary goals I've worked hardest on, and the strategies offered here are the ones that I have found to be most helpful to me personally and have been proven in research studies as well.

As you'll see, we know that one of the best ways is to always have water in front of you whenever and wherever you're seated—at work, at the dinner table, relaxing on the couch, at the movies, or enjoying a cool lemonade on a hot day on your porch.

The PMS three pounds

During your premenstrual phase, you may gain one to five pounds, partly because your body retains water, sodium, and chloride (because of an increase in the hormone progesterone), and partly because you are hungrier and eat more than usual. You may feel bloated, but don't think that by drinking less fluids you'll be less bloated. Continue to drink plenty of liquids, including water and juice, and drink fewer alcoholic and caffeinated beverages. Your body will eliminate any fluids you don't need. Exercise can help, and so can some over-the-counter PMS medications. Within a few days you'll be back to normal.

Think of drinking fluids as a way of preventing thirst, rather than as a response to it, and begin to adopt some of these strategies to increase your fluid consumption:

- Begin every day with a glass of water or fruit juice, in addition to any caffeinated drink you may have.
- Drink a beverage between and at every meal.
- Be prepared. On hiking and walking trips, have more water than you plan to drink on hand if you will not be near a clean water source.
- Take a fresh container of water with you whenever you go out in the car and replenish it as needed.

- A good strategy when you're traveling by car, and one my children love, is to keep plastic bottles full of water in the freezer. As you're traveling, the ice melts and the water stays cold.
- Have an extra glass of cold water or another beverage in the afternoon when you begin to slow down.
- If you like cold water, keep a pitcher of it in the refrigerator.
- If you don't like plain water, drink flavored still or sparkling bottled water. For variety, flavor your water with citrus fruits such as lime and lemon, or puree some pitted watermelon and add sparkling water to it.
- Keep a selection of canned or bottled juices, with no sugar added, in the refrigerator.
- Vegetables and fruits put through a juicer pack plenty of vitamin power. If you have a juicer, try to use a variety of vegetables and fruits in your drinks.

WHAT SHOULD WE DRINK?

It's possible to get optimal fluid intake from a variety of delicious and refreshing sources. Certainly water is the best, most plentiful, and cheapest fluid. However, there are many other options.

Is all water created equal?

The definitions of various kinds of water can be confusing. Here is a brief look at some of the choices:

Public water
Town and city water is usually surface water from reservoirs, lakes, and rivers. In the United States most of our public supplies of drinking water are safe. If your drinking water comes from a public source, it has probably been treated to rid it of contaminants, usually with a disinfectant such as chlorine.

Fluoridated water

Fluoridated water helps prevent dental cavities by making the mineral surface of your teeth harder to dissolve by the acid left from bacteria in dental plaque. Early fluoridation is the most beneficial, starting at birth and continuing until you get your permanent teeth between the ages of 11 and 13.

Although some skeptics claim that fluoridated water causes bone cancers, research has proven the safety of fluoride in water. It is now added to about half the drinking water in the United States, usually in the amount of 1 part fluoride for every 1 million parts water, and the result has been a 50 to 70 percent reduction in cavities.

Private water

Private water is usually groundwater from a well or a spring, and it is generally not cleansed or decontaminated. If you have a well or use spring water, I would suggest that periodically you get the water tested for bacteria or contaminants, as it's hard to say when environmental changes have occurred. Ask your town's health inspectors for guidance in having your water tested. Or you can call the Environmental Protection Agency hotline or use their website, both listed in Resources.

Bottled water

Water from most private and public sources in the United States may look and taste different from place to place, but for the most part it's not harmful. A lot of women ask me if there is an added benefit in drinking bottled water. There are two main types of bottled water: filtered, and water that comes from a natural spring, which usually is labeled mineral water. The filtered water typically does not have any minerals because they have been filtered out. The mineral water usually has trace amounts of minerals such as calcium, magnesium, and salts. Which is best to drink? It all depends on your taste buds.

Home filtration systems

Many people ask me about home water filtration systems. The first thing you should know is that the EPA does not certify or endorse water filtration systems. On their website, the agency cautions that "some people use home water filters to improve taste, smell or appearance of their tap water, but it doesn't necessarily make the water safer or healthier to drink. Additionally, all home treatment devices require regular maintenance. If the maintenance is not performed properly, water quality problems may result."

If you decide to buy a water filtration system, shop around. Most systems use carbon filters, which seem to be useful in removing chlorine, heavy metals such as mercury, and organic contaminants. Other options are "reverse osmosis" filters and distillation systems that filter out contaminants.

If you know that your water supply is safe, and the primary purpose of the filter is to improve the taste of your water, why not buy a simple carbon filter system that can be used in a pitcher and replaced periodically?

Other options for hydration

The healthiest choices are listed first.

Juice

My children love juice. In fact, they prefer it to water. We have fresh orange juice in the refrigerator, and when one of them is thirsty, we simply serve them up a glass of the healthy, nutrient-rich drink.

Drinking juice is a wonderful way to help maintain good hydration. Today you have such a wide range of choices among fruit and vegetable juices, from prune to vegetable blends, from apple to mango, to say nothing of smoothies and combinations you can create yourself. Just make sure you read the label carefully—avoid juices high in sugar, especially added sugar.

Milk

Milk, especially reduced-fat milk, is high on the list of nutritious drinks. It is an important source of calcium and vitamin D, both crucial for growth, strong bones, and strong teeth. If you like milk—and not everyone does—and are not lactose intolerant, I recommend that you drink a glass or two of low-fat milk every day. You will find more information about milk in Chapter 7.

Caffeinated beverages

Caffeine is a natural stimulant found in many common foods and beverages such as coffee, tea, and chocolate. Over the years, there have been a number of studies to determine whether caffeine is bad for you.

During the 1970s and 1980s, research findings appeared that were contradictory. Broad-scale media coverage of some of the studies led to further confusion about the effects of caffeine, particularly on women's health.

Recent, more thorough, research has been conducted which demonstrates that caffeine, taken in moderation, does not have any adverse effects.

- *Coffee:* Drinking more than a few cups of coffee a day has been associated with headaches, trembling, increased heart rate, and insomnia. But each person is different, and your experience should tell you what your own tolerance is for coffee. If you are jittery, having indigestion or problems sleeping, think about how much coffee you drink—perhaps it's too much.

  My personal recommendation is that you drink no more than four cups a day. One study has shown that more than that may increase your risk of heart disease and could be harmful to your bones. Drink coffee in moderation, and do not drink it late in the day.

- *Tea:* I have to admit that I am a tea drinker, and if I don't get my cup of tea in the morning, I am useless. I drag, I get a headache, and I have no motivation. I have been known to fantasize about my cup of tea. I usually have only the one cup—a mixture of Earl Gray and English Breakfast, and I like it with a little bit of honey and some milk.

  I am personally thrilled that, in completed and ongoing studies, scientists have found numerous health-promoting compounds in tea. Both black and green teas contain polyphenols, which have been shown to have properties that are antioxidant, antiviral, anticancer, and antibacterial. (Polyphenols are also found in red grapes, kidney beans, prunes, raisins, red wine and, yes, coffee!)

Antioxidants help prevent heart disease by inhibiting the oxidation of the "bad" cholesterol, LDL. Green tea, at least in the strong concentrations used in several studies, has also been found to kill cancer cells but leave healthy cells untouched. There are studies now underway that will reveal still more about the health-related attributes of both coffee and tea, but until these studies are completed and there is a more definitive understanding of the effect of both of these substances on human beings, my recommendation is to drink both tea and coffee in moderation.

• *Soda Pop:* Soda pop is an old-fashioned expression for a beverage that we can now call by its real name, "empty calories." The only redeeming feature of soda is that it is a fluid. Soda contains sugar, usually in the form of high-fructose corn syrup (a simple sugar); very often caffeine; and flavoring, most of it imitating natural flavors but completely artificial in composition. Sugar-free soda is sweetened with aspartame or saccharine, both non-nutritive sweeteners. They may be safe, but they are synthetic, and they have a chemical aftertaste. I encourage you to avoid them.

If you do drink soda pop, do so in moderation: no more than one a day, if possible. People who drink pop for the carbonation as much as for the flavor find that adding fruit juices to sparkling mineral water or even to seltzer produces a refreshing beverage that eliminates artificial flavors and sweeteners and that tastes more like the real thing—food.

What about alcoholic beverages?

Alcoholic beverages have been around almost as long as humans have. Alcohol is used as medicine, as part of religious ritual, and for enjoyment. Instinctively, we have always known that alcohol is good for us, but it is only recently that we have begun to understand why this is so. Moderate amounts of alcohol can reduce stress, reduce the risk of stroke (probably by lowering risk of blood clots), and reduce heart disease by increasing HDL cholesterol. Beer is more filling and "foodlike" than wine, and it contains some of the B vitamins, which may help reduce heart disease.

Moderation is the key word when drinking alcohol: no more than one drink a day for women. Greater use of alcohol (and any use greater than moderate is excessive use) increases risk of some kinds of cancer, especially rectal cancer, and has been linked with increased bone loss and other health problems.

If you are not already drinking eight cups of fluid a day, I urge and encourage you to do so. To get into the habit, you may have to make the conscious decision, on a daily basis, about what to drink and when and where to drink it. Think about your daily calendar and establish a timetable for regular hydration that suits you best.

Once that routine is in place, you'll begin to notice the changes that being well-hydrated can make in the way you look and feel. Your skin will be clearer, and it will glow. Your digestive system will improve and work more efficiently. Your body will feel more resilient, you'll exercise with more enjoyment, and you'll have more energy for everything you do.

CHAPTER 4

Grains

The Whole Truth

❖

Grains are among our earliest cultivated foods. Since the rise of agriculture almost 10,000 years ago, grains have also been our single most essential food. Whole societies rose and fell based on their ability and subsequent failure to provide grain for their people. Whole societies have subsisted almost entirely on grains; some still do. Today, wheat, rice, and corn are the most important food crops worldwide. And yet, paradoxically, the value of grains in the human diet has been the subject of intense debate in recent years, and no other food group has received more controversial press—good and bad—than grains.

Some of the science behind the controversy is easily understood, other aspects are quite complex because there are complicated biochemical issues involved, as you will see.

CARBOHYDRATES:
THE HALF TRUTH, THE WHOLE TRUTH

The bad rap for grain has been fueled by the popularity of the get-thin-quick schemes promoted in a number of diet plans, all based on the simplistic idea that a high-protein, low-carbohydrate diet will help you *Lose Weight Fast!* and keep you *Skinny for Life!* and maintain your health *Forever!*

The half-truth

The claim that carbohydrates, especially those from grains, make you fat is partly right. Over the last twenty to thirty years, the American food industry has inundated us with hundreds of thousands of palatable but highly refined, high-calorie products made from grain, and they unquestionably contain large amounts of carbohydrates. These carbohydrates *will* make you fat.

For many Americans, such foods have become dietary staples, and there is no doubt that their consumption, coupled with an increasingly sedentary lifestyle, has been the greatest contributor to the escalating problem of obesity in our society. The foods I am talking about are doughnuts, cookies (especially "fat-free" cookies), white pasta, refined, sweetened breakfast cereals, white bread, bagels, white rice, sports bars, snack foods, and candies of all kinds. These are the foods that are harming our health and making us fat.

The whole truth

What has been left out of the discussion is the *kind* of carbohydrates we eat and the quantities in which they are consumed. Here's where these diet plans are wrong. The truth is, not all carbohydrates make you fat. Genuine whole-grain brown rice, true whole-wheat bread, and real whole-grain cereals such as oatmeal do not contribute to obesity. The reverse is true: these foods and other whole grains help to promote health and reduce our risk of developing a number of chronic diseases.

The Food Guide Pyramid recommends that we eat six to eleven servings of grains every day, and many of us do. (As you will see later in the chapter, I recommend eating six to eight servings a day.) But Americans get few whole grains in their diet. We may eat a bagel for breakfast, have brown bread (which usually does not have 100% whole wheat listed as the first ingredient) for lunch, and for dinner eat a large bowl of pasta, with snacks in between, often made of refined grains. Where are the whole grains?

I am not recommending draconian measures, nor do I believe we must excise all highly processed grains from our lives. I think there is a place for every kind of food in our diet, including a limited quantity of refined grains. We all enjoy the occasional dish of pasta or slice of pizza or a flaky, buttery croissant. But if the only grains we eat are refined, we have not only put ourselves on the road to obesity (or pushed ourselves a little further down that road), but we have cheated ourselves of culinary pleasure. It may come as a shock to many Americans, but whole grains are delicious!

WHAT'S IN WHOLE GRAINS?

Whole grains contain much more than just carbohydrates. They are a source of fiber, which comes in several forms, vitamins, minerals, and phytochemicals. Most important, whole grains taste very good, and, because they are filling, they help to regulate satiety so that you don't overeat.

Fiber

Fiber is what gives plants their structure, and it is found in all foods that originate in plants. Although it is a type of complex carbohydrate, fiber is not a nutrient because it cannot be digested or absorbed into the bloodstream and converted into energy. Instead, it is excreted. But fiber does aid in digestion, and it also may offer protection against certain diseases.

There are two main types of fiber:

Insoluble fiber (cellulose, hemicellulose, or lignin) does not dissolve in water, as its name implies. It is also known as "roughage" and can be found in whole-wheat products such as cereals and breads, in wheat bran and corn bran, and in vegetables such as potatoes and green beans. Here are some of the ways insoluble fiber works in the body:

- It absorbs water (but doesn't dissolve in it) and makes you feel full.
- It can work as a natural laxative by stimulating the intestinal walls to contract and relax (peristalsis), causing food to move through the digestive tract.
- It may help prevent or relieve digestive disorders or diverticulosis.
- It adds bulk and softness to stools, promotes regularity, and prevents constipation.
- It moves waste through the colon quickly so harmful substances don't linger in the intestines and come in contact with the intestinal lining.

Soluble fiber (gums, mucilages, or pectins) dissolves in water. It is found in oat bran and barley and in fruits and legumes. Among its properties:

- It appears to lower cholesterol because pectin binds, or adheres, to fatty substances, prevents their absorption by the body, and promotes their excretion as waste.
- Soluble fiber reduces risk for heart disease.
- The pectins in some soluble fibers form gels with water and make you feel full.
- Soluble fiber helps regulate the body's use of sugars.

A chart listing the fiber content of many different foods is on page 241.

Carbohydrates

Carbohydrates, the body's main source of energy, are classified as either simple (sugars) or complex (starches). The basic simple sugar is a compound that has six carbons linked together. The most common simple sugar is glucose. Complex carbohydrates are composed of chains of many glucose units (polysaccharides: *poly* = many, *saccharides* = sugar) linked together. They are found in grains, such as rice and wheat, and in potatoes and other vegetables, such as legumes.

Glucose supplies much of the energy used by the body's cells, including our brain cells, which use it as their main energy source. When we eat complex carbohydrates, the chains of glucose are broken down during digestion into individual glucose units that are absorbed through the walls of the small intestine into the bloodstream and transported throughout the body. With the help of insulin and glucose transporters, blood glucose is brought inside the cells, especially muscle cells, where it is used as energy.

Small amounts of glucose are not used immediately, but stored in the liver and muscles and kept in reserve for use when the body's blood glucose levels fall. As an example, if you have gone without food for an unusually long period of time or have exercised vigorously, your cells can call on the glucose stored in your muscles and liver for an immediate source of energy.

Proteins and fat

Grains are not a significant source of fat unless, of course, fat is actually added to the grain during cooking—croissants, cakes, muffins, and doughnuts come to mind. Any fat that is contained within the grain is mostly monounsaturated or unsaturated and therefore is health-promoting. Protein content depends on the type of grain and whether it is a whole grain, with the germ intact, or refined, with the germ lost during processing.

Phytochemicals

Flavonoids, polyphenols, and isoflavones (see Chapter 5), all phytochemicals found in whole grains, act as antioxidants and are health-promoting. Most if not all of these phytochemicals, which are located in the germ of the grain, are lost when the grain is refined.

Vitamins and minerals

Grains are also an important source of vitamins and minerals, such as beta-carotene, B vitamins, vitamins C, A, and E, and selenium, zinc, copper, iron, and other trace minerals. These are naturally contained inside the whole grain, with most of the nutrients in the germ. When grains are refined, most of their nutrients are lost.

Diseases attributed to deficiencies of these nutrients were noted only after large-scale refinement of grains began. For many decades, from the mid-1800s through the 1920s, scientists believed that the diseases resulted from toxins in rice. During the late 1920s and through the 1930s, scientists discovered that nutrients had actually been removed from the grain during the refining process. As a result, in 1940 Congress passed legislation mandating that grains be "enriched" with iron, thiamin, riboflavin, and niacin to add back the nutrients to the levels that naturally occur in whole grains. In 1996, Congress enacted further legislation that grains must be fortified with folate, a B vitamin considered essential in the prevention of neural tube defects. Folate has also been cited as a means of regulating homocysteine, an amino acid associated with the risk of having a stroke or heart attack. (See page 67.)

WHOLE GRAINS CAN REDUCE THE RISK OF CHRONIC DISEASE

Scientists, nutrition professionals, and a growing number of people interested in healthy foods have all recognized the essential, positive value of whole grains in our diet. This same community also understands that refined and overprocessed grains are unhealthy to the point of being nutritionally negative. The main paradox in the controversy over grains is that refined grains can actually *cause* the same diseases that whole grains help to prevent.

Now, after years of research and many studies, we understand some, although not necessarily all, of the ways in which whole grains can help reduce the risk of disease.

A healthy heart

Numerous studies have demonstrated the positive relationship between intake of whole grains and the reduction of heart disease. The exact reasons for

Glycemic index / Glycemic load

The glycemic index quantifies the rate at which carbohydrates from a particular food enter the bloodstream and raise blood glucose.

Foods with a high glycemic index enter the bloodstream quickly, raise blood sugar levels fast, and produce an inflated insulin response. Foods with a low glycemic index enter the bloodstream more slowly, raising blood sugar levels less quickly, and producing a moderate insulin response. Foods are ranked from 1 to 100, with 100 being the highest in terms of blood glucose response.

It is important not to look at any single food in isolation. You must consider everything you eat in context and understand your meal patterns to get an idea of the overall glycemic index for your total diet. A small potato will not contribute to obesity and diabetes, but an extra-large portion of French fries with a hamburger on a white bread bun and a large soda pop, eaten on a regular basis, will.

Glycemic load is a factor that is often overlooked and is as important as glycemic index. It is the sum of the glycemic index of a particular food plus the amount of sugar actually contained in the food.

Foods with both a high glycemic index, which enter the bloodstream quickly, and high sugar content will elicit a high (unfavorable) insulin-spike response. Such foods are considered to have a high glycemic load.

Foods with a high glycemic index but only a small amount of sugar will not induce the insulin-spike response and are considered to have a low glycemic load. Such foods, which contribute fiber and quality carbohydrates, are found in whole grains as well in as some fruits and vegetables, and they are important to a healthy diet.

For example, when you eat a carrot, which has a very high glycemic index, it enters your bloodstream quickly. However, because it does not contain much carbohydrate, the carrot does not have a

oad and will not trigger a large increase in your blood
e is true for some other fruits and vegetables, with the
otatoes, which have both a high glycemic index and
as do white breads and soda pop.

this beneficial effect are difficult to pinpoint, but many scientists believe that in large part it is due to the high fiber content of whole grains—especially the soluble fiber in oat bran, barley, and fruits and vegetables—which helps lower LDL cholesterol in several ways.

- Bile acids in the intestines are produced from cholesterol. Soluble fiber binds with some of the bile acids and transports them out of the body during excretion, which has the effect of reducing the amount of blood cholesterol.
- Bacterial by-products that result from the digestion of soluble fiber in the colon inhibit production of cholesterol in the liver.
- Some research indicates that people who habitually eat foods high in fiber tend to replace fattier foods with those high in fiber. However, even when the consumption of fatty foods remains unchanged, most studies, including the Nurses' Health Study, have shown that there is an independent positive effect of fiber on reducing the risk of heart disease.

The Nurses' Health Study and coronary heart disease (CHD): One study on fiber and grains showed a range of intake from a low of 11 grams to a high of 23 grams per day. Women in the highest range had a reduced risk of CHD. Among the various food sources of fiber, only dry breakfast cereal was strongly associated with reduced risk of CHD.

Another interesting finding was that the lower risk of CHD associated with increased whole-grain intake could not be completely explained by the fiber, folate, vitamin B_6, and vitamin E contained in grain. There may be some other elements in grains that are health promoting—perhaps undiscovered phytochemicals.

Glycemic Index Chart

Foods that contain carbohydrates are classified on a scale
refers to the speed at which the carbohydrate in the foods
stream as glucose.

High glycemic index foods are classified as above 74
Intermediate glycemic foods = 51 to 74
Low glycemic foods = 50 or less

HIGH GI	INTERMEDIATE GI	LOW GI
White and rye bread	Whole-wheat bread	Old-fashioned oatmeal
Water crackers	Muffins	Buckwheat groats
Refined, sugary cereal	Croissants	Pumpernickel bread
White bagel	Pita bread	Stone-ground WW bread
White rice	Popcorn	Milk
Carrots	Ice cream	Yogurt
Potatoes	Brown rice	Cheese
French fries	Granola bars	Peanuts
Rutabaga	Beets	Sponge cake
Broad beans	Banana	Oranges, grapefruit
Dried dates	Raisins	Peaches
Soda, sports drinks	Pineapple	Pears
Jelly beans, sugar candies	Papaya	Apples
Corn chips	Mango	Grapes
"Fat-free" cookies	Orange juice	Apricots
Corn flakes	Sports bars	Chocolate
Graham crackers	Most cookies	Lentils
Pumpkin	Corn	Baked beans
	Oatmeal, quick	Soybeans
		Egg pasta, plain pasta

Note: Glycemic index varies with brands. Generally, the higher the added sugar content and the more refined, the higher the glycemic index.

Decreasing your risk of cancer

High-fiber diets are also associated with a decreased risk of colon cancer, although once again the reasons why are not entirely clear.

Several studies have supported the theory that whole grains are protective against cancer, particularly colon and gastric cancer. One possible explanation is that fiber dilutes, binds, and helps with rapid removal of potential cancer-causing agents from the colon. Certain vitamins and minerals as well as phytochemicals may all act as antioxidants. Another possibility is that people whose diets are high in fiber and low in animal proteins can develop health-promoting bacteria in the small intestine. When these particular bacteria ferment, it has the effect of lowering pH (the acid base balance), which has been associated with a decreased risk of colon cancer.

I believe that the overwhelming evidence supports the recommendation that, to reduce the risk of developing cancer, women should consume a diet high in a variety of fiber-rich foods.

Exercise and blood glucose

Exercise uses up the energy stored in the body's cells, especially muscle cells. Muscle cells become very sensitive to insulin, a hormone whose primary purpose is to control the movement of glucose from the bloodstream into cells, and to glucose transporters whose sole purpose is the transport of glucose. When you exercise, a series of biochemical responses enhances the action of insulin and glucose transporters and helps remove glucose from the bloodstream easily.

The more sedentary and overweight you become, the less efficiently your insulin and glucose transporters work, and this can lead to diabetes. Even if you have type 2 diabetes, exercise can make insulin and glucose transporters much more sensitive so that it is possible for some people to reduce their dependency on drugs and keep their blood sugar under control.

The Nurses' Health Study

The Nurses' Health Study is an important ongoing federally funded study initiated in 1976 by scientists at the Harvard Medical School. A group of 121,700 female nurses, 30 to 55 years old, was selected. The study was set up originally to look at the health effects of the birth control pill, but very quickly, the scientists realized that they were working with an enormously rich resource for studying lifestyle issues such as diet, exercise, body weight, smoking, and their effect on diseases, health, and longevity.

Nurses were chosen because, although they are the same as other working women in terms of childbearing, eating, and smoking, their professional training and experience require them to be organized, accurate, and observant, and thus easier to study and follow. Over 90 percent of the women are still in the study!

Since 1976, these women have had regular health evaluations, with particular focus on the possible links between various aspects of nutrition, health, and disease. As part of their evaluations, the nurses answer detailed questionnaires regarding their nutrition habits, their blood, urine, and even toenail clippings are collected. The study has already yielded more than 250 scientific publications, and is still in progress.

Keeping your glucose under control

There are two ways in which high-fiber foods help prevent and manage diabetes: first by helping control weight, and second, because soluble fibers trap nutrients and delay their transit through the GI tract, slowing glucose absorption and helping prevent a glucose surge in the intestine. By slowing down the digestive process, soluble fiber may also help to control blood sugar, reducing the need for insulin or other medication.

The Nurses' Health Study examined the relationship between foods rich in carbohydrates and fiber and type 2 diabetes. In trying to determine how factors such as fiber and glycemic load influence the development of diabetes over time, scientists found that women who ate more foods with high glycemic indexes *and* who had a diet with a high glycemic load were much more likely to develop type 2 diabetes.

Researchers also looked at several specific foods to determine their association with diabetes. What they found was that cold breakfast cereal and yogurt were protective against the disease and that cola drinks, white bread, white rice, French fried potatoes, and other cooked potatoes had positive associations with diabetes; that is, they contributed to the disease.

Maintaining a healthy weight

Weight gain is a major risk factor for type 2 diabetes, perhaps the most important factor. Whole grains can make a difference. High-fiber foods take longer to chew, they require more water to digest, and they reach a higher volume in the stomach than the same amounts of processed carbohydrates. The result is that whole grains fill you up and increase satiety, which means you eat less. High-fiber foods are digested more slowly. They empty out of the stomach at a more gradual pace, delaying a sense of hunger, so that you eat less frequently. Finally, high-fiber foods tend to be lower in fat than processed foods.

In the mid- to late 1980s, Tufts University did a series of studies on diet, exercise, and glucose control in people who were at risk for type 2 diabetes. In our earliest studies, we found that when refined carbohydrates were replaced with whole grains, several things happened. At first, people in the study felt full very quickly and had a hard time finishing their meals; they lost weight over the first few days. Early in the study, some of the participants experienced gas and intestinal discomfort, which improved as soon as they adjusted to the increased fiber their diets. Mostly, they felt as if they were eating carloads of food, even though they weren't eating any more calories.

Whole grains and other high-fiber, high-volume foods and their relationship to weight loss are the subject of a number of studies now underway. We can expect more useful information from this research that will help us achieve and maintain a healthy weight and help to stem the epidemic of obesity.

GI health

If you eat a low-fiber diet, as many Americans do, you are at much greater risk for constipation and diverticulosis (bulges that develop in weakened areas of the colon). Cultures with high fiber intake do not have these problems. Taken with ample fluids, high-fiber foods help to prevent hemorrhoids and diverticulosis. These foods reduce constipation and allow indigestible waste and bacteria to pass more quickly through the large intestine. However, anyone with diverticulosis should talk with a doctor before undertaking a high-fiber diet. Foods such as berries and the skins of certain fruits can cause problems. For instance, the small seeds of berries can become imbedded in the diverticula (small pouches in the colon) and get infected.

SMART STRATEGIES FOR EATING
MORE WHOLE GRAINS

Whole grains and soy products (Chapter 8) are two crucially important food categories, and too many of us are unfamiliar with them. We all know about whole-wheat bread (although we may not eat it), and most of us have heard that oat bran is a beneficial addition to baked goods and cereals, and we may, every now and then, eat buckwheat pancakes.

But how many of us can remember the last time we ate barley, brown rice, spelt, bulgur wheat, or a wheatberry salad, whole-wheat couscous, true whole-grain bread, or any of the other wonderful grains listed later in this chapter?

Like most people, I love grains—all types: breads, rice, cornbread, biscuits, barley. I am lucky, though, because I have always enjoyed whole more than refined grains. Through graduate school and beyond, I have eaten whole-wheat and cornmeal pancakes several times a week for breakfast. I always look for good, dense whole-wheat or multigrain bread for sandwiches for lunch.

And when we eat rice at home, it's almost always short-grain brown rice. If I'm in a rush and revert to white rice, I always feel that I am eating tasteless starch—I'm so used to the nutty, sweet brown rice! And if I am served white bread instead of whole grain, I feel as if I'm getting "air" bread.

I do realize that this preference for whole grains is an acquired taste not necessarily shared by everyone. When you begin to reduce the amount of refined, highly processed grains in your diet and start to eat more whole grains, do so gradually. Rapid and large increases in whole grain consumption can cause gastrointestinal discomfort. Notice that I said "reduce" refined grains, not "cut completely."

In one large study of women's health and diet, researchers found that, on average, the ratio of refined to whole grains in participants was 20:1, when it should be 1:1. As you can see, there is a lot of room for improvement in most women's diets.

Grain Glossary

Terms that appear on grain labels

Enriched (sometimes wrongly used interchangeably with *fortified*): with breads and cereals, meaning that five nutrients have been added: thiamin, niacin, folate, riboflavin, and iron. Nutrients are added to meet a specified, established standard for a particular product. Thiamin, folate, and riboflavin are added in amounts that are nearly equal to or greater than those originally contained in the product before processing. Iron is added to help prevent iron-deficiency anemia.

Fortified: referring to a food with nutrients added that it did not originally contain. For example, many breakfast cereals are fortified with vitamins and minerals that don't naturally occur in grains.

Refined: having the coarse parts of a food removed. The bran, germ, and husk are all removed when wheat is refined into flour, leaving only the endosperm.

Unbleached flour: tan-colored endosperm flour with texture and nutrient values similar to white flour.

Wheat flour: flour made from wheat; includes white flour that has been refined.

White flour: endosperm flour, bleached and refined to maximize softness and whiteness.

Whole grain: contains all but the husk of a grain milled in its entirety but not refined.

Whole-wheat flour: whole-grain flour that is made from whole-wheat kernels.

Other important terms relating to grains

Bran: fiber-rich protective outer coating around the kernel, similar in function to the shell of a nut. It retains the B vitamins and trace minerals found in the plant.

Endosperm: inner part of the grain, the majority of the edible part of the kernel. It contains starch/carbohydrates and proteins, and a small amount of vitamins and minerals.

Germ: seed that grows into a wheat plant, very rich in B vitamins, trace minerals, and some protein. It resides on the inner part of a grain next to the endosperm.

Gluten: elastic protein found in wheat that gives dough its structure and cohesiveness.

Husk (also called chaff): outer, inedible coating of a grain. It surrounds the bran.

How many total servings of grain should you get every day?

The Food Guide Pyramid recommends consuming six to eleven servings of grain overall every day. Unless you exercise vigorously and for a long duration on a regular basis, I recommend that you do not eat the full number of servings suggested. All grains, whole or refined, are relatively high in calories, and they add to the glycemic load, discussed above. This combination contributes to obesity.

A combination of three to four whole-grain and two to three refined-grain servings per day is a good balance. You will be able get enough fiber and other health-promoting benefits from the whole grains, but still have room for some of the refined grains. I strongly believe that at least half to three-quarters of the grains we eat each day should be whole grains.

Serving sizes for grains

The serving sizes I use in my books are based on the Food Guide Pyramid.

For grains, the following amounts count as one serving and contain 60 to 100 calories each: ½ cup cooked grains (oatmeal, brown and white rice, pasta, cereals, wheatberries, barley, cornmeal, corn grits); 1 slice bread; ½ small bagel; ½ English muffin; 1 small dinner roll; 5 saltine-type crackers; 1 ounce pretzels; 1 cup cold cereal.

These serving sizes are much smaller than those most people and most restaurants usually serve. For example, a typical bagel you'd buy at a local deli can easily be four to five servings of grain. A "normal" serving of rice or pasta should actually be counted as two servings.

Beginner's luck

If you have been accustomed to eating a diet that includes very few whole grains and not much fiber, the way to begin is slowly. Avoid the intestinal discomfort experienced by the subjects of the Tufts study, whose entire daily intake of refined grains was replaced by whole grains in a single day. Instead, add one or two different whole grains a week to your daily intake and reduce the refined grains by a slightly greater amount. Within a month, you should be eating about three or four servings a day of whole grains, or at least half your grain intake. That way, your digestive system will have time to adjust to a new biochemical experience, and your palate will have time to sample a number of different grains, which you can select and reject and substitute at will.

Here are more ways to get the best out of grains:

- Think about the times during the day when you eat refined grains: breakfast cereal, sandwich at lunch, a candy bar snack, white rice or semolina pasta for dinner, TV snack later on. Then think about where you can substitute a whole grain for a refined one: oatmeal for breakfast, real whole-grain bread for your sandwich, whole-wheat crackers for a snack, brown rice with your dinner. Look at the sample menus at the end of this chapter to get an idea of the whole grains you can substitute, then try them, and try some of the recipes in this book.
- Spend some time in one or two well-stocked health-food stores to acquaint yourself with the range of whole-grain products available. Talk to store employees; most of them are knowledgeable, and they are always happy to provide information, advice, and encouragement if you feel somewhat timid about trying a new food.
- Buy from health-food stores that get a lot of traffic—their inventory is fresher, a point to consider if you are buying whole-grain products or any other foods.
- Depending on where you live and how insistent you and other customers are on the subject of whole grains, some supermarkets are beginning to sell them. Use what you have learned from shopping in health-food stores to buy whole-grain products in these larger venues.
- Unless you know you will be using them soon, or unless you have a lot of freezer or refrigerator space, don't buy large quantities of whole grains at one time. Because they are not refined and are not processed with preservatives, whole-grain products tend to retain their natural oils and can spoil if left too long on the shelf.

- Some whole grains—barley, bulgur, kasha, and quinoa—cook as quickly as refined grains. Others, which are equally delicious and add to the pleasure and variety of what you eat, take longer to cook—brown rice, wild rice, whole wheat berries, whole kernel hominy, among them. Plan your meals accordingly.
- If you don't have the time to cook a particular grain for dinner or lunch, cook it in the morning or the night before. Most grains will keep well if they are packed in tightly covered vessels or refrigerator bags and stored in the refrigerator.
- Substitute barley, spelt, and brown rice for white rice or pasta in soups.
- Read labels carefully. The words *whole wheat* and *whole rye* should appear at the beginning of ingredients lists for breads and cereals. The words *wheat flour* don't mean *whole wheat*. Most white bread flour is made from wheat that's been refined and processed.
- Seek out products that contain a significant amount of fiber: 2 to 4 grams per slice of whole-grain bread, and 2 to 5 grams per serving of whole-grain cereal.
- In baking, use whole-wheat flour for at least half the total flour amount.

THE WHOLE GRAINS

The list that follows will give you a brief look at the wonderful variety of delicious whole-grain products that are available—most of them in supermarkets and health food stores, or through mail order sources or websites (see Resources for a few starting places). Organic whole grains are usually preferable, but not a bottom-line necessity.

Major grains

Wheat: One of the two earliest cultivated foods. Wheat is made into flour, cereals, breads, cakes, and many other products, and is also available in its most basic form as **wheatberries,** which have become a new favorite of mine. **Wheat bran** is added to cereals and sometimes to baked goods.

Bulgur, which is steamed wheatberries, and *semolina,* which is durum wheat milled and made into pasta and couscous, are other wheat products. *Spelt, kamut,* and *farro* are early forms of wheat that can be purchased as berries and are very tasty.

Barley: The second earliest cultivated grain. It is available whole (virtually inedible) and pearled (delicious). Cooks quickly. Use in soups, risottos, salads—any way you would use rice.

Rice: Half the world's population uses rice as its main source of carbohydrates. It is made into hundreds of products, from flour to noodles to vinegar. Although there is an almost infinite number of varieties of rice, it is the different kinds of brown rice that interest me: *long-grained brown* and *short-grained brown rice, brown Basmati,* and *brown Texmati* (an American version of Basmati). All can be bought in supermarkets. Astonishingly versatile.

Corn: One of the world's great staple foods. From those kernels on the cob to popcorn to polenta, it is delectable. Like every other food-for-profit, corn has been hybridized and genetically altered to infinity. *Stone-ground cornmeal,* preferably organic, still retains the germ and hull of the kernel, making it healthier than degerminated cornmeal, although both kinds are enriched. *Grits,* like cornmeal, are ground from the kernel of either white or yellow corn, the grits being the coarser part of the meal left after the finer cornmeal is sifted out. Grits are a Southern specialty (and a Saturday morning favorite at our house) and most flavorful and healthy when they are stone-ground. Stone-ground grits are mostly available by mail order (see Resources). The fine white quick grits, packaged by major food producers and available in supermarkets, have virtually no flavor or food value whatever, other than as a source of carbohydrates.

Whole-kernel hominy, or *posole,* is the whole corn kernel treated with unslaked lime or wood ash. The ground hominy kernel becomes *masa ha-*

rina, used for tortillas; the whole kernel is either cooked and canned, or dried and sold for soups, stews, and other long-cooking dishes. Cooked dried posole is chewy and flavorful, reminiscent of corn, but not sweet. Dried packaged posole can be bought in some health-food stores and Hispanic groceries, and is now packaged by Goya Foods as well.

Buckwheat: Milled as flour, it is familiar to us as an ingredient in breakfast pancakes and blini. Less familiar but very delectable is *kasha,* or *roasted buckwheat groats,* which are sold packaged in supermarkets or in bulk in health food stores. Kasha cooks quickly and can be substituted for rice in dishes where its earthy flavor will not overwhelm the other ingredients. My family loves it for winter breakfasts with some nuts and fruit added.

Oats: Used as a cereal and an ingredient in baked goods, such as breads, scones, and, of course, those cookies. *Rolled oats,* which can be bought in any grocery or supermarket nationwide, cook very fast. *Steel-cut oats,* which are organic and chewier, cook more slowly, but are well worth the wait.

Rye: Used mostly as bread flour in rye and pumpernickel breads. When purchasing rye bread from a bakery, be sure to ask whether whole-grain rye flour is one of the ingredients. Most of the rye grown in this country is used for rye whiskey.

Lesser-known grains

Quinoa is native to South America—a mild-tasting grain, packed with high-quality protein, and quick-cooking. Available packaged and organically grown, even in supermarkets.

Wild rice is actually a grass. Once harvested exclusively by Native Americans in Minnesota, it is now cultivated in California. It has a chewy texture, earthy flavor, and is still quite expensive. It is available in health food stores, gourmet food shops, and through mail-order sources. Good in combination with brown rice, wonderful in pilafs, salads, stuffings, and as an accompaniment to main course proteins.

MENUS

The following menus show that you can have whole grains, fiber, protein, and fruits and vegetables no matter what your daily calorie intake is.

1,600-Calorie Classic Mixed Menu

MEAL	CALORIES	FIBER	CALCIUM
BREAKFAST			
½ cup old-fashioned oatmeal, dry	148	3.7	19
½ cup 1% milk	51	0	150
½ cup fresh blueberries	40	2	9
8 oz. fresh orange juice	112	3	27
SNACK			
1 apple with skin	81	4	10
8 oz. vanilla yogurt	200	0	350
LUNCH			
Turkey sandwich:			
2 slices whole wheat bread	138	3.8	40
2 slices turkey breast	46	0	2
1 tbsp. mayo	100	0	0
1 oz. slice cheddar cheese	114	0	204
2 leaves iceberg lettuce	4	0.6	8
Sliced tomato (¼ whole tomato)	7	0.4	5
Carrot sticks (1 medium carrot)	31	2.2	19

(continued)

DINNER	CALORIES	FIBER	CALCIUM
Salad:			
1 cup romaine, shredded	8	1	20
Chopped tomato (¾ whole tomato)	19	1	1
Chopped carrot (1 medium)	31	2.2	19
1 cup sliced cucumber	14	1	14
3 oz. salmon	127	0	14
2 tsp. olive oil	83	0	0
½ cup broccoli, boiled	22	2.3	36
½ cup cauliflower, boiled	14	1.7	10
⅔ cup brown rice	170	2	0
SNACK			
2 cups plain air-popped popcorn	61	2.4	1.7
Totals:	**1,621**	**33.3**	**959**

2,000-Calorie Classic Mixed Menu

MEAL	CALORIES	FIBER	CALCIUM
BREAKFAST			
2 large eggs, scrambled with milk	202	0	86
2 slices pumpernickel toast	160	4.2	22
1 tbsp. butter	108	0	4
8 oz. orange juice	112	3	27
SNACK			
8 oz. plain yogurt	140	0	400
1 cup fresh strawberries	45	3.4	21
LUNCH			
Bean and cheese burrito:			
7–8" flour tortilla	114	1.2	44

1 oz. jack cheese	106	0	212
2 chopped leaves iceberg lettuce	4	0.6	8
Chopped tomato (½ whole tomato)	12	0.8	2
½ cup black beans	113	7.5	23
⅓ cup brown rice	85	1	0
1 cup cantaloupe pieces	56	1.3	18
DINNER			
4 oz. cooked haddock fillet	126	0	48
1 cup broccoli, boiled	44	4.6	72
1 baked potato with skin	220	4.8	20
1 tbsp. sour cream	26	0	14
8 oz. 1% milk	102	1.8	300
SNACK			
1 medium pear	98	4	18
1 oz. cheddar cheese	114	0	204
Totals:	**1,987**	**38.2**	**1543**

2,000-Calorie Vegan Menu

MEAL	CALORIES	FIBER	CALCIUM
BREAKFAST			
¾ cup cream of wheat	100	1.3	38
1 tbsp. honey	64	0	2
½ cup fresh raspberries	30	4.2	14
8 oz. fresh grapefruit juice	96	0.2	22
SNACK			
Mango	135	3.7	21

(continued)

LUNCH	CALORIES	FIBER	CALCIUM
Spinach Salad:			
2 cups raw chopped spinach	24	3.2	112
½ cup raw firm tofu	183	2.9	258
½ cup kidney beans	103	4.5	69
2 oz. roasted sesame seeds	320	8	560
2 tbsp. Italian dressing	140	0	4
Navel orange	60	3.1	52
DINNER			
Rice and beans with sautéed vegetables:			
⅔ cup brown rice	170	2	0
½ cup black beans	113	7.5	23
½ cup chopped raw onion	30	1.4	16
1 clove garlic	4	0	5
½ cup yellow summer squash	18	1.3	24
½ cup zucchini	14	1.3	12
Chopped tomato (1 whole)	26	1.4	6
1 tbsp. olive oil	124	0	0
SNACK			
8 oz. chocolate soy milk	110	3.1	300
½ cup edamame	127	3.8	131
Banana	105	2.7	7
Totals:	**2,096**	**55.6**	**1,676**

I find it fascinating that over the last twenty-five years grain consumption has increased, and yet fiber consumption has not changed at all—it still remains low. At the same time there has been a dramatic increase in the number of people who are overweight. I do not think that these statistics are coincidental.

Our culture must take action to reverse this trend. I firmly believe that

Americans can reduce the intake of refined grains, increase whole-grain consumption, and stop the rise in chronic disease associated with a refined, low-fiber diet. The women I have worked with who have made this change in their own eating habits have seen remarkable results—and they love the new foods and flavors they are discovering.

CHAPTER 5

Fruits and Vegetables

The Dream Team for
Health and Pleasure

❖

In the summer, my family and I spend as much time as we can at the farm in New Hampshire where my husband grew up and his parents and brother still live. Tom, my brother-in-law, is an organic farmer, and he supplies most of the local community with fresh, delicious fruits and vegetables through the summer and long into the fall. It is a gorgeous spot, and I feel especially privileged to spend time on the farm. Not only is it beautiful, but my children get to spend time with their grandparents, and we always eat the best because of the abundance of fresh, delicious food.

I can't imagine a meal without at least some fruits and vegetables. They taste so good—and most of them are low in calories, and they can reduce your risk of getting so many diseases—that you'd think everyone would eat at least as much of these foods as they need, if not more. But in the United States, only a quarter of the population eats the five to nine servings a day that's recommended. We have a long way to go.

FRUITS AND VEGETABLES:
MORE THAN JUST VITAMINS

We don't yet know *all* the reasons fruits and vegetables are so healthful. We do know that they supply the majority of the essential vitamins and minerals we need to live.

In general, we receive our largest supply of vitamin C, vitamin K, vitamin A (through beta-carotene), folate, and potassium from produce. Vegetables and fruits also contribute some of the body's store of magnesium, calcium, and other trace minerals. While vegetables and fruits are generally low in calories, they do supply us with carbohydrates, which are an important energy source for the body.

Another component of fruits and vegetables (and of whole grains, too) is fiber, which is a significant factor in good digestion and an aid in reducing cholesterol and in utilizing glucose for energy. Studies have shown that people who increase their consumption of fruits and vegetables tend to decrease the amount of processed foods and saturated fats, with a direct and beneficial effect on their health.

Both simple and complex carbohydrates are found in vegetables and fruits. Carbohydrates are the primary source of the body's fuel and provide half of its energy, as discussed in greater detail in Chapter 4.

Fruits and vegetables also provide compounds called phytochemicals (*phyto* = plant) that at present are under intensive research to discover their potential for preventing disease. Many of the phytochemicals and vitamins and minerals in vegetables and fruits act as potent antioxidants in our bodies, helping to destroy the free radicals that cause cell damage.

Antioxidants

A diet high in vegetables and fruits is considered to be the most effective way to stabilize free radicals. Free radicals are unstable, or chemically unbalanced, molecules that are formed as part of the body's normal metabolic processes when the cells use oxygen to produce energy. Pollution, tobacco smoke, radiation, and other environmental factors can also create free radicals.

Whatever their cause, free radicals attempt to stabilize themselves by taking particles from other molecules, which themselves become free radicals and in turn steal particles from other nearby molecules. This chain reaction can cause large-scale damage to the cells and may result in a number of life-threatening diseases.

Antioxidants donate an electron to the unstable free radical without becoming unstable themselves, thus halting the chain reaction. The body is equipped with a supply of its own antioxidants—a built-in repair system—but they are insufficient in themselves and must be replenished from the antioxidants in foods: vitamin A from beta-carotene, alpha carotene, vitamin C, vitamin E, some minerals, and phytochemicals.

Phytochemicals

Phytochemicals are naturally occurring compounds found in plants. They serve a protective function within the plants themselves and have, in a number of instances, been shown to protect the human body against heart disease and cancer, among other chronic diseases associated with aging. Fruits and vegetables, along with whole grains and soy, contain a range of phytochemicals that are now being studied singly and in combination in an effort to understand more of their health-promoting properties.

Lycopene is one of the best-studied phytochemicals. It is present in abundance in tomatoes, and research has shown that men who eat large amounts of tomatoes, especially cooked tomatoes, have a reduced risk of developing prostate cancer. We believe that lycopene may also act as a preventative in other types of cancers. Two other phytochemicals, lutein and zeaxanthin, which are present in yellow, orange, and dark green leafy vegetables, are usually found together and are believed to reduce risk of macular degeneration, the leading cause of blindness in the elderly.

FRUITS AND VEGETABLES REDUCE THE RISK OF CHRONIC DISEASE

The nutrients and phytochemicals contained in fruits and vegetables participate in a series of biochemical processes that have the effect of sustaining or improving your health. A diet rich in vegetables and fruits can help reduce your risk for certain forms of heart disease, hypertension, cancer, cataracts and macular degeneration, diabetes, constipation and diverticulosis, and osteoporosis.

A blueberry a day . . .

Blueberries and two other plant foods have recently been studied for their phytochemical power. Tufts scientist James Joseph and his colleagues investigated the possibility that spinach, strawberries, and blueberries could reverse the mental, nerve, and muscle decline in mature rats. The investigators split the rats randomly into four groups, and each group was fed one of the four following diets for a period of eight weeks: a regular diet, or a diet supplemented with spinach, strawberry, or blueberry extract.

The investigators found that all three groups of older rats eating the extract-supplemented diets had an increase in important chemicals in the brain and improved cognitive function, but those given blueberry extract showed the greatest increase. The rats on the blueberry extract diet showed the most improvement in their ability to swim through a water maze (a test for cognitive function) and to walk on a rod or plank and hang onto a wire (demonstrating improved motor function).

These results have not yet been replicated in humans, but the study, one of numerous research projects now underway, does show us how important it is to eat your fruits and vegetables!

Within days of the release of these results to the national media, fresh blueberries, which were out of season at the time, began appearing in every produce market across the country. Naturally, I bought some, and I've been serving them regularly ever since.

Phytochemicals identified in fruits and vegetables

FOOD SOURCES	PHYTOCHEMICAL	FUNCTION IN THE BODY
Citrus fruits	Limonene Phenols Terpenes	• Increase enzyme production to help excrete carcinogens • Antioxidants • Reduce carcinogens • Reduce formation of malignant tumors (tamoxifen and taxol, both used to treat breast cancer, are terpenes)
Colorful fruits and vegetables such as carrots, sweet potatoes, spinach, broccoli, cantaloupe, pumpkin, apricots, mangos Vitamins: folate, vitamin C, vitamin K	Carotenoids including beta-carotene, alpha-carotene, beta-cryptoxanthin	• Antioxidants • May reduce risk of cancer, heart disease, and age-related vision problems
Leeks, chives, onions, garlic	Allyl sulfides	• Increase enzyme production to help excrete carcinogens • May impede reproduction of tumor cells
Cruciferous vegetables such as broccoli, cabbage, kale, Brussels sprouts, and cauliflower Vitamins: folate, vitamin C, vitamin K	Sulforaphane Dithiolthiones Indoles Isothiocynates	• May prevent cancer by helping the body convert a potentially harmful form of estrogen into a harmless form

Grapes, strawberries, raspberries	Ellagic acid	• Guards against in tobacco and pollutants
Legumes such as green beans and peas, also cherries	Phytosterols Isoflavones Saponins	• Interfere with cell reproduction in GI tract, delaying cancer growth • Block estrogen activity in cells
Apples, celery, cranberries, grapes, black and green tea, red wine, onions, oregano	Flavonoids	• Antioxidants, thereby reducing risk of heart disease by decreasing oxidized LDL cholesterol as well as cancer
Yellow, orange, and dark green leafy vegetables	Lutein and zeaxanthin (these are actually carotenoids, usually found together in foods)	• Antioxidants • Lower risk for macular degeneration
Fruits such as blueberries, prunes, raspberries, grapes	Caffeic acid Ferulic acid	• Stimulate enzyme production to make carcinogens harmless
Tomatoes (need some fat in order to absorb lycopene)	Lycopene	• Reduces risk for prostate cancer • May reduce different cancers in women

Antioxidants and your heart

There are abundant reasons why eating a diet rich in fruits and vegetables will reduce a woman's risk of heart disease. Fruits and vegetables provide antioxidants that can stabilize free radicals inside the arterial walls. When low-density lipoproteins (LDLs) become oxidized by free radicals they are much more likely to form plaque and to adhere to any micro injuries within the arterial walls. Research shows that vitamin C may act in concert with vitamin E to keep LDL cholesterol from becoming oxidized, which may in turn reduce plaque in the arteries and lower the risk for heart disease. The antioxidant properties of these two vitamins are also thought to help prevent the oxidative damage to arterial walls caused by tobacco smoke or by a diet high in saturated fats.

Homocysteine and heart disease

An exciting new field of research has focused on homocysteine, an amino acid which, in high levels, may contribute to the risk of heart disease and which has also been implicated in other conditions such as colon cancer (see below), Alzheimer's disease, miscarriages, birth defects, osteoporosis, strokes, and presbyopia (aging of the eyes).

Elevated levels of homocysteine occur in the body as a result of low intake of B vitamins—especially folate, B_6, and B_{12}—but can also be associated with loss of estrogen, smoking, stress and anxiety, and with a diet high in animal proteins.

The good news is that there is a direct relationship between the amount of folate in the diet and homocysteine levels in the blood: the more folate you take in, the lower your homocysteine levels. Folate is found in high concentrations in green leafy vegetables and citrus fruits and juices. Recently, flour used in baked goods has been fortified with folate, not to prevent heart disease, but to reduce neural tube defects in the unborn children of pregnant women. The overall consequence of folate fortification is that blood homocysteine levels in the population as a whole are dropping. We believe this will reduce heart disease as well.

There are now more than fifteen studies underway, supported by the National Institutes of Health, to determine the benefits of reducing homocysteine levels. Until the results are in, it makes sense to eat a varied diet that is low in animal protein and high in fruits, vegetables, and grains.

Fruits and vegetables influence blood pressure

About one third of the American adult population is estimated to have hypertension. Vegetarians are more likely to have lower blood pressure than non-vegetarians, probably because they eat more of the fiber and minerals, such as potassium, magnesium, and calcium, which are known to reduce blood pressure.

Numerous studies have tried to identify the "active" ingredient in vegetarian diets that reduces blood pressure, but these attempts have generally been unsuccessful. Potassium supplement trials have lowered blood pressure to some extent, but magnesium, calcium, and fat modification have produced little or no effect.

The Dietary Approaches to Stop Hypertension (DASH) Study

Now there is solid scientific research showing that eating fruits and vegetables can reduce blood pressure. The DASH Study is an ongoing, multi-center research project located at Harvard to study the effects of dietary patterns on blood pressure. The goal of one of the first research projects out of the study was to find a diet that retained the blood pressure benefits of the vegetarian diet, while still including enough meat products to make the diet palatable and acceptable to non-vegetarians.

DASH concluded that blood pressure can be lowered significantly in older adults by a diet that includes low-fat dairy products (2.7 servings per day), is high in vegetables and fruits (eight to ten servings a day—more than the Food Guide Pyramid recommends), and is low in fat (about 30 percent a day). People following this diet showed an average decrease in their systolic (top number) pressures of 5.5 points and a drop of 3 points in their diastolic pressures, compared to the control group, which ate an average American diet.

Fruits and vegetables can protect against cancer

Cancer is the blanket term we use to cover a number of diseases—there are over 100 different types. The characteristic they all share is that they arise when cellular DNA is altered and cells begin to multiply out of control and form tumors.

Some of the causes of cancer are genetic, some are environmental, and many are due simply to old age. Cancer and its causes, prevention, and cure are being researched in literally thousands of studies.

Diet is one of the major fields of research in the prevention of cancer. Epidemiological studies have linked consumption of a diet high in fruits and vegetables with a low incidence of a range of cancers that are associated with cell damage from free radicals. What is clear from these studies is that eating a variety of fruits and vegetables, and a variety of different whole foods in general, is an important way to protect against cancer.

Folate, which has been shown to reduce homocysteine levels and lower the risk for heart disease, may play a similar role in lowering the risk for colorectal cancer. Consistent observations show that the largest increases in cancer of the colon and rectum come when folate intake is low and alcohol consumption is high. High folate intake also seems to reduce the risk for cervical, lung, stomach, and esophagus cancer, although the associations aren't as strong as with colorectal cancer.

Scientists are now investigating the mechanisms by which low folate levels increase the risk of cancer. One avenue of research may show that when folate intake is low, DNA becomes more susceptible to damage, and the natural defense systems of the cells may be compromised.

Phytochemicals and healthy eyes

Cataracts are the thickening and clouding of the eyes' lenses, with older individuals being at highest risk. Damage to the lens can result from oxidative stress as a by-product of ultraviolet exposure. Some studies that show such damage can be decreased by eating a variety of foods high in antioxidant nutrients such as vitamins C and E and carotenoids. Supplements of vitamins C and E may also lower the probability of developing cataracts for older people.

Macular degeneration is another disease characterized by loss of vision. It is the most common cause of blindness in older people. The role of diet as a means of preventing or impeding the progress of macular degeneration is now the subject of a number of studies. The National Eye Institute is conducting a long-range Age-Related Eye Disease Study, which will eventually give us more definitive information than we now have. A diet rich in antioxidant nutrients has been shown in some studies to correlate with a lower rate of the disease.

The phytochemical lutein, a carotenoid found in leafy green vegetables, is also found in the macula, the region of the eye that is responsible for visual acuity. Macular pigment density is thought to be inversely related to risk of age-related macular degeneration, and it has been found that macular pigment can be increased by increasing lutein and zeaxanthin from spinach and corn in the diet.

Improving glucose control

There are 15 million Americans with type 2 diabetes, and its incidence has tripled during the last forty or so years. Unchecked diabetes can cause serious complications such as heart disease, stroke, blindness, kidney failure, and amputations. A strong genetic predisposition may be a factor in type 2 diabetes, but lifestyle plays a large role as well, especially for women who are obese and sedentary.

New research is now demonstrating what we have known instinctively all along: a diet high in processed foods and simple sugars and low in fiber can be instrumental in the development of the disease in older adults. A diet high in fruits, vegetables, and whole grains reduces the risk of developing diabetes by about 30 percent.

Fruits and vegetables for a healthy gut

Eating a diet rich in fiber, especially soluble fiber, can minimize constipation and diverticulosis. (See Chapter 4 for a more detailed discussion of fiber.) The fiber found in many fruits, vegetables, and some cereal grains together with water helps to make the stool larger and softer, and stimulates peristalsis, the muscle contractions that move matter through the GI tract. People from cultures whose diets are high in plant-based food have a very low rate of both constipation and diverticulosis.

Better bones

Recent research shows us that vitamin C, vitamin K, potassium, and magnesium are important nutrients to improve bone health and reduce risk of osteoporosis. Women who consume a diet rich in these nutrients (a diet rich in fruits and vegetables) have higher bone density on average than women who eat less of these foods.

Vitamin C is necessary for collagen production, the first phase of bone formation. Vitamin K is also necessary for the formation of collagen through the production of osteocalcin, a protein critical for bone formation. One recent Harvard University study showed that women who ate an average 110 micrograms per day of vitamin K had a 30 percent reduction in the incidence of hip fractures. Half a cup of green leafy vegetables supplies us with more than 110 mg of vitamin K.

Magnesium contributes to the mineralization, or hardening, of bones. Studies have shown a relationship between high potassium intake and denser spines and hipbones in women. It is possible that this is because potassium helps maintain the proper acid base balance in the blood, which means that the body doesn't need to withdraw calcium from the skeleton for this purpose.

An important finding in all these studies is that the benefits derived from these nutrients do not seem to be available from vitamin and mineral supplements. They are to be had by eating foods rich in these nutrients—green leafy vegetables, cruciferous vegetables, bananas, citrus fruits, and mangoes.

Future findings

This is an exciting time for the scientists who are studying the roles that diet and dietary patterns play in the prevention and reduction of chronic disease. We already know some of the health-promoting qualities provided by the vitamins, minerals, and phytochemicals found in fruits and vegetables, and we know that there are many other combinations of these components yet to be discovered and evaluated.

SMART STRATEGIES FOR EATING MORE FRUITS AND VEGETABLES

Recently, I was in North Carolina to give a presentation. One night I had dinner in the hotel dining room, and I could hear the gentleman at the

Why don't I just take a vitamin pill?

There's no doubt that you can take a multi-vitamin-mineral supplement to increase your body's levels of antioxidant vitamins as well as folate. But vitamin pills or other nutritional supplements are not an adequate substitute for eating an abundant quantity and variety of fruits and vegetables. First, there is the sheer pleasure to be had from eating good foods. And from a nutritional standpoint, there are many other compounds in fruits and vegetables that contribute to optimum health and that cannot be replicated in the right balance and amounts in a pill, because we still don't know them all.

Having said that, there is accumulating research showing that supplements may provide additional or potential benefits for reducing heart disease, improving immune function, and reducing the risk of cataracts and macular degeneration. Choose a basic multivitamin supplement that contains close to 100 percent of the recommended levels. Make sure that the supplement contains vitamins C, folate, B_6 and B_{12}. You may need a separate supplement for vitamin E, up to 400 IU a day is recommended. There is no evidence that taking more that 400 IU a day of vitamin E has any additional benefit for these diseases.

table next to me talking to the waitress. First he ordered soup, then meat—of course. When the waitress described his options for side dishes, instead of one of the three vegetables she mentioned, he wanted potato, no other vegetables at all. The soup's fine, but not a *single* green or yellow vegetable? This is not uncommon. We should be *asking* for vegetables, even if the waiter doesn't offer them. Nine times out of ten the kitchen has something—broccoli, spinach, carrots—so even if vegetables are not on the menu, request them.

Functional foods: Too much of a good thing?

Functional foods is a term referring to foods that have been form-ulated, either by food manufacturers or through genetic modi-fication (see Chapter 11), to provide special nutritional benefits by preventing or reducing the risk of disease and improving overall health. Functional foods are actually an updated version of enriched or fortified foods, such as milk, juices, and cereals, to which vitamins and minerals have been added, a practice that began as early as the 1940s.

Now, in addition to vitamins and minerals, food manufacturers are adding other biologically active components to their products: phytochemicals, which I discuss in this chapter and in Chapter 6, and herbal supplements, such as ginkgo biloba, St.-John's-wort, echi-nacea, and others. These substance-enhanced products may or may not deliver the benefits their manufacturers claim for them. For the most part, their capability for promoting health has not yet been proven conclusively.

Beyond their unproven benefits, there are two issues that concern me and other nutrition scientists:

- These substances are not regulated for purity, nor are the amounts of them that are added to various food products monitored.
- We still don't know how these herbs and even certain phyto-chemicals will interact with other medications and how they will affect people whose health is at risk.

I have no doubt that certain functional foods hold great potential for maintaining and improving our health, such as fruits and vegeta-bles that contain naturally occurring phytochemicals. And vitamins and minerals that have been added to foods in regulated amounts have already been proven effective in preventing disease. But until further research has been conducted into the practice of super-loading food products with large amounts of vitamins and herbs, my recommendation is to eat whole foods as they are. If you wish to take an herbal supplement, do so separately and only after discussing it with your doctor.

Food manufacturers are not shy about promoting the presumed health benefits of their functional foods. These are typical products: snack bars, cereals, and packaged smoothies and other drinks.

How many portions should I eat?

National guidelines recommend that we eat between five and nine fruits and vegetables a day. I agree with these guidelines but urge you to work toward the higher rather than the lower end—eat seven to nine portions a day. Not only that, but I strongly encourage you to eat—regularly, if not on a daily basis—citrus fruits and leafy dark green vegetables, as well as those that are deeply colored in oranges, reds, and yellows. They are the ones that tend to be the most nutritious.

Eat three or four portions of fruit every day

- Start each day with fruit—either juice or served with yogurt or combined with cereal.
- Treat yourself to a new flavor by trying a fruit you haven't eaten before, or eat a new variety of a familiar fruit. New types of apples, plums, grapes seem to appear daily on the produce stands.
- Treat yourself to an old favorite—the first local organic strawberries or blueberries, early crisp apples, the clementines that herald the holiday season.
- Use your good senses of smell, sight, and touch when you buy fresh fruits so they are at their peak when you eat them.
- Fruits are a good high-energy afternoon snack, and many of them come prepackaged by nature in handy portable portions.

- Don't buy more fresh fruit than you and your family can eat or store for a few days.
- Keep bags of frozen fruits in your freezer to have on hand whenever you need them.
- Puree fresh or frozen fruits to use as sauces for ice cream, yogurt, and other desserts.
- Puree fruit with tofu, soy milk, or yogurt and ice to make low-fat smoothies or cool, refreshing lassi (see page 237 for recipes).
- Keep a supply of canned juices in your refrigerator for a quick pick-me-up.
- Stimulate your senses; think about the fruit before you serve it. How will you cut it up and set it out so that it appeals to your taste buds, eyes, and sense of smell?
- Dried fruit, eaten in moderation because of its high sugar content, is a satisfying snack.
- Add juice or a combination of juices to chilled seltzer or mineral water for a cool summer drink.

Eat four or five portions of vegetables every day

- When dining out, order a vegetable you haven't eaten before or one prepared in a way that might not have occurred to you. If you like it, find out where to buy it, how to prepare it. Try to eat a different new vegetable once or twice a month.
- When dining in, bring your restaurant experience home. Look through books in the library or a bookstore, search the Web. Clip interesting "home-style" recipes from newspapers and other publications and use the recipes included in this book.
- Have meal-of-the-month parties with friends and include two or three vegetable dishes in each menu.
- Small vegetables, such as cherry and grape tomatoes, baby carrots, Kirby cucumbers, radishes, and white button mushrooms, and finger foods such as celery, endive, and edamame are handy snacks.
- Visit nearby farmers' markets to get the freshest produce. Some of the small farms that supply the markets may grow heirloom vegeta-

bles and fruits or other produce unfamiliar to you. Ask questions; farmers are always knowledgeable about what they grow and eager to share that knowledge.

- Buy vegetables in manageable amounts, and don't buy more than you can eat or store for a few days.
- When you travel, whether in the United States or abroad, visit food stores and outdoor farmers' markets to see how and what other people are growing and eating.
- Vegetables taste better if they are not overcooked. Quick-cooking methods, such as steaming and stir-frying, preserve nutrients and flavor.
- One way to get kids to eat root vegetables is to make them into a rich stew. I often do this on winter weekends, when I combine all the vegetables left over from the week—butternut and acorn squash, potatoes, turnips, carrots, mushrooms, and barley. The kids love it, and we get at least two meals out of it.

Serving sizes for fruits and vegetables

The serving sizes I use in my books are based on the Food Guide Pyramid.

For fruits, the following amounts count as one serving and contain 80 to 100 calories each: 1 medium whole fruit, such as apple, peach, orange, nectarine; 1 small banana; ½ grapefruit; 1 cup diced melon; ¾ cup juice; ½ cup berries or grapes; ½ cup diced, cooked, or canned fruit; 2 tablespoons raisins; ¼ cup dried fruit.

For vegetables, the amounts listed count as one serving and contain 10 to 40 calories each: ½ cup cooked or raw vegetables; 2 cups leafy raw vegetables; ¾ cup vegetable juice; ¼ cup avocado; ½ small potato; 3 tablespoons salsa; 1 cup sprouts.

GETTING THE BEST

I get so much pleasure from eating fruits and vegetables that sometimes I find it difficult to believe others don't share my enthusiasm. In summer

But what about the sugar?

Many women tell me they love to eat fruits and vegetables, but they have read or been told that they shouldn't enjoy these foods because of their high sugar content. It is true that the main energy source in fruits and vegetables is carbohydrate.

But carbohydrates are not bad when they come naturally from produce, which provides some of the most important nutrients to sustain life. All the fruits and vegetables that provide us with vitamins, minerals, and phytochemicals that help prevent disease also contain sugar or carbohydrates that become sugar, and sugar translates into calories. But, eaten judiciously, these are calories that count toward health, not the empty calories found in soda pop, candy, and other sugar-filled foods, which contribute to disease.

Instead, I encourage you to enjoy a rich variety of fruits and vegetables every day at every meal.

when I see my children at the family farm sitting in the berry patch eating handfuls of luscious berries, or when we pick three or four of the ripest vegetables from the garden for our evening meal, I know that we are experiencing a little bit of heaven here on earth.

But, like most of you, I don't live in or even near heaven most of the year, and, like you, I have to find ways to feed my family the delicious food they want and need.

Seasonal pleasures *plus* a world of choices

When I can, I prefer to buy seasonal produce. There is something about eating fruits and vegetables in season that satisfies our human desire for change and at the same time allows us to feel that we're part of the natural cycle. Produce tastes better in season, and of course it's usually cheaper as well.

Organic or non-organic

I've often been asked whether I recommend buying organic produce instead of fruits and vegetables grown with commercial fertilizers and pesticides. What we know is that there is not much difference between the amounts of vitamins and minerals found in organic and non-organic foods. However, when there is a choice, I always try to eat organic vegetables and fruits. I think they taste better, and as you will read in Chapter 11, I think there are good environmental and political reasons to do so. But when organic produce is not available or too expensive or looks wilted and tired, I don't buy it. Local produce, whether organic or not, always seems best to me because we can eat it so soon after it's been harvested that its flavor and nutrients are at their peak, and at the same time we can support our local farmers.

Buy selectively

Most of us live near two or three stores that sell produce—supermarkets, greengrocers, small food stores, and farm stands. Whenever you shop for fresh fruits and vegetables, if you have the time I suggest you take a critical look to see who has the best looking fresh food, who carries local produce in season, and who sells good organic seasonal vegetables and fruits.

When I am going to buy fruits and vegetables at the supermarket, I usually spend most of my shopping time in the produce section, and I consider it time well spent. My daughters complain because I'm not fast enough, but I dispatch them to other sections of the store, where they can pick out the rest of the items on our shopping list. I need the time to smell and touch and look.

And so should you. Use your judgment, your creativity, and your experience when you shop for fruits and vegetables. Select produce that is whole and intact, and that does not show bruises, cuts, insect holes, decay, or mold.

The ABCs of fruits and vegetables?

One of my favorite strategies, when I'm trying to think of new foods for my family to eat, is to look at a list of fruits and vegetables. Reading the names spurs my interest and reminds me of what we haven't tried in a long while and what my children have never eaten and might enjoy.

Fruits: many varieties of apples, apricots, Asian pears, avocados, bananas, berries of all kinds, cantaloupes, casabas, carambolas, cherimoyas, cherries, clementines, cranberries, crenshaws, currants, dates, figs, grapefruit, grapes, guavas, honeydews, kiwis, kumquats, lemons, limes, loquats, lychees, mangoes, nectarines, oranges, papayas, passion fruits, peaches, pears, persimmons, pineapples, plums, pomegranates, prickly pears, raisins, quince, starfruit, tangerines, and watermelons.

Vegetables: artichokes, arugula, asparagus, bamboo shoots, beets, beet greens, bok choy, broccoli, broccoli rape, Brussels sprouts, cabbage, carrots, cauliflower, celery, celery root, chard, Chinese broccoli, collard greens, corn, cucumbers, daikon, eggplant, endive, hearts of palm, kale, kohlrabi, leeks, lettuces, lima beans, lotus root, mushrooms in profusion, mustard greens, okra, onion, parsnips, peas, bell peppers, hot peppers, potatoes in rainbow colors, pumpkin, radicchio, radishes, rhubarb, rutabaga, scallions, seaweed, shallots, spinach, sprouts, summer squash, winter squash, string beans, sweet potatoes and yams, taro root, tomatillos, tomatoes, turnips, turnip greens, water chestnuts, watercress, wax beans.

Fresh, frozen, canned, or dried?

Although we've all been told for years that fresh is best—and often it is—we don't always have that choice. Fresh may not be fresh: It may be wilted or wrinkled or too early or too late to be at its prime. Or it may not be available when you want it.

Fortunately, we always have available to us foods that have been processed—that is, frozen, canned, or dried—which in many instances are as nutritious as fresh food. The reason is that food producers usually process food as soon after harvest as possible, preserving its nutrient value and much of its flavor. Very often, the technology is brought to the harvest site, and processing begins immediately while the food is at its freshest.

Drying foods, especially fruits, fish, and meat, is one of the earliest forms of food preservation. Among vegetables, tomatoes, mushrooms, all manner of beans, peas, pepper flakes, and a wide range of herbs are widely available.

Dried fruits are a kitchen staple. They range from apples to cherries to pineapples to raisins and cranberries and strawberries. They are delicious, they make convenient and nutritious snacks, but they should be consumed in moderation because of their high sugar content.

I always love the season I'm living in. Right now, it's spring, and in our family we look forward to May because our local farmer has the best asparagus, and we eat it almost every day for a month—along with as many other seasonal fruits and vegetables as we can find. But much as I delight in spring, it is not necessarily my favorite season. I can't wait for summer, when the farm stands and markets near us seem to burst with ripeness and color. And I always look forward to fall, when we can buy Brussels sprouts on the stem from farmers' markets, and then in early October we go apple-picking in Vermont orchards. Winter root vegetables are so beautiful to look at and so marvelous to eat that I live in happy anticipation of the vegetable roasts and stews I'll be making in December and January.

CHAPTER 6

Calcium and Vitamin D

Strong Bones for Life

❖

Every time I walk down the street and see a woman hunched over from spinal fractures, every time I get a call from a woman who is suffering from osteoporosis, my resolve to help women—and to look after my own bones—becomes stronger.

I began researching exercise, nutrition, and bone health in women at Tufts when I was 23 years old. Since that time, a new world has opened up. We now know that we can strengthen our bones, whatever our age. We have learned that osteoporosis is a preventable disease, and that if you already have it, you can treat it. The most important thing you can do is to start right now—whatever your age—to make sure that your bones last a lifetime.

Osteoporosis is a devastating disease that can leave a person frail, deformed, depressed, disabled, and in pain. Osteoporosis is characterized by loss of bone density, which leads to fragile bones that are susceptible to fracture. One in three women can expect to suffer from the disease in her lifetime. In fact, one in two women and one in eight men over 50 will have an osteoporosis-related fracture in their lifetimes.

In the United States today, 10 million people already have osteoporosis, and 18 million more have low bone mass, putting them at risk for osteoporosis. A woman's risk of dying from the complications of a hip fracture are greater than her risk of developing breast, cervical, and uterine cancer combined.

Osteoporosis is a completely silent disease. You cannot feel yourself losing bone. Only after you have suffered from a fracture are you aware that the disease has crept up on you. Hip, spine, and wrist are the bones most susceptible to fracture, although any bone can fracture from the disease. Wrist fractures in women in their mid-fifties have recently been noted as an early sign of osteoporosis.

By about age 20, the average woman has accumulated 98 percent of her skeletal mass. Building strong bones during childhood and adolescence and maintaining those bones into later life is the best defense against developing osteoporosis.

A comprehensive program that can help prevent this disease includes a diet that is rich in calcium and vitamin D, plenty of exercise—especially weight-bearing and strengthening exercises—and a way of life that excludes smoking and excessive use of alcohol. Some women may need to take medication to prevent or treat osteoporosis.

Strong Women, Strong Bones, my previous book, presents all the latest information about osteoporosis. If you are at risk for the disease, I encourage you to read the book and to use the Resources at the back of this book.

CALCIUM: THE FUNDAMENTAL NUTRIENT FOR STRONG BONES

Calcium is the most plentiful of the seven major minerals in our bodies. There is over a pound of calcium in the human body, and it performs a number of critically important functions.

Calcium and our bones

Ninety-nine percent of the calcium in our bodies is in our bones and teeth. From childhood to early adulthood our bones visibly grow and change, but adult bones too acquire and lose minerals and are continuously being re-modeled. Calcium is needed for optimal remodeling and the maintenance of strong bones.

The calcium in our bones also serves as a storehouse of calcium for the rest of the body. When blood calcium falls too low, the body withdraws calcium from the bones, returning it when blood calcium rises too high.

Blood calcium

Although only 1 percent of the body's calcium is in the bloodstream, it is essential to life. Research has shown that calcium is related to hypertension: The mineral switches on a protein that transmits messages from the surface of a cell to its interior. Among these messages are some that help to preserve normal blood pressure.

Blood calcium is essential for regulating muscle contractions and blood clotting, it helps to conduct nerve impulses, and it works to activate a number of hormone reactions.

HOW MUCH CALCIUM DO WE NEED?

Calcium's relationship to several diseases is the subject of current investigation. For example, research has already shown that people with moderate to high blood pressure can reduce their blood pressure by eating a diet that contains ample amounts of calcium, especially when that diet includes plenty of fruits and vegetables. Dietary calcium may also play a role in diabetes and some cancers, and it has a possible connection to lowering blood cholesterol.

But by far the most important way calcium works to prevent disease is in reducing the risk of osteoporosis. Calcium is the major nutritional factor contributing to healthy bones.

Since 1975, more than 135 scientific papers have been published that describe the connection between calcium intake and bone health, from childhood through old age. This research demonstrates that, depending on age group, a nutritious diet containing 800 to 1,300 mg of calcium per day is

DIETARY REFERENCE INTAKE OF CALCIUM FOR WOMEN AND MEN

AGE	CALCIUM DRI (MG/DAY)
Birth to 6 months	210
6 months to 1 year	270
1 to 3 years	500
4 to 8 years	800
9 to 18 years	1,300
19 to 50 years	1,000
51 to 70 years	1,200
71 years and older	1,200

Source: National Academy of Sciences, 1997

critical for the development of strong bones in childhood and the maintenance of bones as we grow older. The chart above shows calcium requirements at every stage of life.

Calcium in our food

The table on pages 89 and 90 offers a wide range of food sources of calcium. Use the table to estimate the amount of calcium you are getting from food now, then use it as a planning tool to increase your calcium intake, if necessary. Although dairy foods are unquestionably the best source, many others, such as calcium-fortified soy products, juice, and breakfast cereals, provide as much calcium as dairy foods.

Leafy green vegetables, while not as calcium-rich as the "excellent sources," nevertheless contain enough of the mineral to make a difference in your

Medications and osteoporosis

If you have osteopenia (low bone mass) or osteoporosis (very low bone mass), exercise and nutrition are critical, but you will also need to talk to your doctor about medication. The combination of exercise, nutrition, and medication management is by far the best way to reduce your future risk of a fracture.

Luckily we now have more medications from which to choose. The medications listed below are approved by the FDA for the management of osteoporosis. Talk to your doctor about which, if any, would be the best one for you, based on your family and personal medical history.

Estrogen replacement therapy (ERT, numerous brand names)
Alendronate (brand name Fosamax®)
Risedronate (brand name Actonel®)
Raloxifene (brand name Evista®)
Calcitonin (brand name Miacalcin®)

New medications are under investigation, and I suspect that over the next five to ten years we will see more effective treatment for osteoporosis.

overall daily intake. They also provide some of the crucial vitamins, minerals, and phytochemicals the body needs, as well as adding the variety that is the hallmark of any pleasurable meal.

THE CRITICAL COMPANIONS: VITAMIN D AND OTHER CALCIUM ENHANCERS

While calcium is of primary importance for reducing the risk of osteoporosis, other nutrients are necessary as well. Of these, the largest and most crucial contribution is made by vitamin D.

Sources of Calcium in the Diet

EXCELLENT SOURCES 200 MG OR MORE PER SERVING		
FOODS	**SERVING SIZE**	**CALCIUM (IN MG)**
Milk (whole, low-fat, skim)	8 ounces	300
Protein-fortified milk	8 ounces	350
Yogurt (whole, low-fat, non-fat, flavored)	8 ounces	275–325
Protein-fortified yogurt	8 ounces	400–450
Hard cheeses high in calcium: cheddar, Swiss, Edam, Monterey Jack, provolone, Parmesan, Romano, part-skim mozzarella	1 ounce	200–300
Ricotta (whole milk, low-fat, nonfat)	½ cup	250–350
Soy milk (calcium-fortified)	8 ounces	200–300
Soybeans: dry roasted; soy nuts	½ cup	225
Tofu made with calcium sulfate	½ cup	250
Calcium-fortified orange juice	8 ounces	200–300
Calcium-fortified breakfast cereal and fortified snack bars	1 cup	150–600
Calcium-fortified soy beverage	8 ounces	200–300
Salmon (canned, with bones)	3 ounces	200
GOOD SOURCES OF CALCIUM 100–199 MG PER SERVING		
Hard and soft cheeses with medium calcium levels: American, Gouda, Colby, whole-milk mozzarella, feta, Fontina, blue cheese, Camembert	1 ounce	100–199
Milk-based puddings and custards	½ cup	150
Soybeans: green boiled; edamame	½ cup	125

(continued)

Tofu made without calcium sulfate	½ cup	125
Protein-fortified cream cheese	1 ounce	100
Spinach, cooked	½ cup	125
Rhubarb, cooked	½ cup	175
Sardines (canned with bones)	2 sardines	100
Anchovy (canned with bones)	3 ounces	125
MINOR SOURCES OF CALCIUM **25–99 MG PER SERVING**		
Soft cheese lower in calcium: Brie, Neufchâtel, cream cheese (regular, low-fat)	1 ounce	20–50
Cottage cheese (whole milk, low-fat, nonfat)	½ cup	60–80
Ice cream and frozen yogurt (regular, low-fat, nonfat)	½ cup	70–99 (Note: some brands are higher.)
Soy milk (not calcium-fortified)	8 ounces	10

Vitamin D and our bones

Vitamin D acts to strengthen our bones and teeth by increasing the absortion of calcium in the gut and by assisting with the mineralization of calcium in bone. When vitamin D is insufficient in the body, calcium absorption is also sub-optimal, and the symptoms of vitamin D deficiency are similar to those of calcium deficiency: rickets in children, whose weakened bones and muscles cause bowed legs and a protruding abdomen; osteomalacia, or adult rickets, which affects young adult women; and, of course, osteoporosis, or extreme loss of calcium from the bones. Rickets and osteomalacia are relatively rare in the United States, but osteoporosis is on the rise, due to longer life expectancy, sedentary habits, poor nutrition, and detrimental lifestyle factors that harm bone, such as smoking and disordered eating.

What the research shows

The importance of vitamin D in preventing bone loss was shown definitively in a seminal study of calcium supplements undertaken at Tufts University in the late 1980s through the early 1990s by Bess Dawson-Hughes, M.D., and colleagues. The subjects were a group of 389 men and women volunteers (mostly women) over 65, about half of whom were given daily calcium supplements that contained a significant amount of vitamin D, with the control subjects being given placebos.

In following these men and women over the course of three years, the scientists discovered that the volunteers receiving the calcium supplement with vitamin D, which contained 500 mg of calcium and 700 IU of vitamin D, had half the number of fractures as those taking the placebo.

There have been no studies showing that calcium supplementation alone can reduce fractures. Vitamin D is the critical addition to calcium that makes the difference.

How much vitamin D do I need?

The following chart shows your vitamin D requirements. The DRIs are the same for women and men.

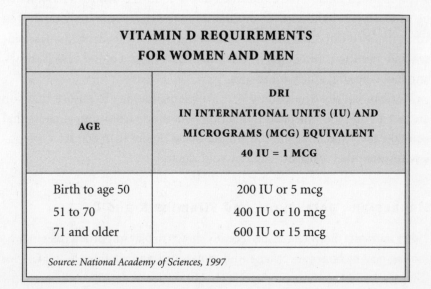

VITAMIN D REQUIREMENTS FOR WOMEN AND MEN	
AGE	**DRI IN INTERNATIONAL UNITS (IU) AND MICROGRAMS (MCG) EQUIVALENT 40 IU = 1 MCG**
Birth to age 50	200 IU or 5 mcg
51 to 70	400 IU or 10 mcg
71 and older	600 IU or 15 mcg
Source: National Academy of Sciences, 1997	

Sources of vitamin D

Vitamin D is readily available, although in relatively few sources.

- Sunshine, one of the best things in life that's free, is a major source of vitamin D. During the spring, summer, and fall, if you spend ten to fifteen minutes a day with your hands and legs exposed to the sun, your body will be able to manufacture as much vitamin D as it needs. In the northern half of the United States, we make little or no vitamin D in our skin during the winter months.
- Milk fortified with vitamin D is another important source.
- Other animal-derived foods: egg yolks; liver; cold salt-water seafood such as salmon, sardines, mackerel, tuna, shrimp, and oysters.
- Fortified cereals.
- Multivitamins and some calcium supplements.

Can I get too much vitamin D?

The answer is yes. Your body stores vitamin D, and when you consume it continuously, either in food or in supplements, in amounts higher than the recommended intake (the established upper limit is 2,000 IU a day), it can be toxic. Hypervitaminosis D, or vitamin D toxicity, occurs only rarely, but when it does it can cause calcium withdrawal from the teeth and bones, nausea and vomiting, and severely harmful effects on the blood vessels, heart, and lungs, among other soft tissues.

Toxicity usually occurs only with supplementation. To ensure that you are not getting too much, add up all the vitamin D from supplements that you take every day. The amount should be no higher than 800 IU a day unless you are otherwise instructed by your doctor.

Magnesium, potassium, and vitamins K and C

Other nutrients that research has recently shown to play important roles in promoting healthy bones are magnesium, potassium, and vitamins K and C. (See Chapter 5 and the chart on pages 244–249 for more detailed information.)

Protect your skin from the sun

For many of us the most natural and pleasurable way to get enough vitamin D is through exposure to the sun. But too much sun can wreak havoc with your skin: age spots, wrinkles, dry skin, and skin cancer are potential risks. Many women have asked me how much sun exposure they should get and how to protect themselves. Here are some guidelines for getting the benefits of sunlight without increasing your risk of skin problems:

- Always protect your face from the sun. Wear a hat or put sunscreen of at least SPF 15 on your face. Nothing will age skin faster than exposure to the sun, and the fragile skin on your face is especially susceptible to sun damage of all kinds, so cover up.
- During the day, when you are outside for 10 to 15 minutes, expose your arms and legs to the sun. This short amount of time is enough for your daily dose of vitamin D.
- If you plan to be in the sun for longer than 15 minutes, cover up your skin with clothing or use sunscreen of at least SPF 15. This holds true even when there is a light haze in the sky, because the sun still can penetrate and cause damage to your skin.
- Protect your eyes by wearing good-quality sunglasses and a hat. The sun's ultraviolet rays can damage your eyes as well as your skin.
- Never allow your skin to become sunburned.
- It's important to talk to your doctor about any changes in your skin, such as new moles, moles that have changed in shape or become discolored, or any other variations in your skin. These changes may be a sign of skin damage from the sun, which can result in skin cancer. Most forms of skin cancer are easy to treat, but they must be caught early!

STRATEGIES FOR GETTING ENOUGH CALCIUM

One of the thoughts that has occurred to me over and over again as I've written this chapter is that all the nutrients we need for developing and maintaining strong, healthy bones come from almost every food category: dairy, vegetables and fruits of all kinds, whole grains, legumes, soy products, fish, fowl, meats—everything except fats and sugars. If we follow up on the belief that whole, unprocessed foods are the cornerstone of our health and of our pleasure in eating, we can achieve the goal of getting enough calcium from food quite easily.

Calcium

- Take the time to familiarize yourself with some of the calcium values for foods that you like (see the table starting on page 89), then use those foods in your diet, throughout the week, throughout the year. I am notorious in my family for adding yogurt to a lot of dishes because it has a pleasant tang of its own and yet adapts well to other flavors. I add it to soups, sauces, baked goods, salad dressings, and serve by itself with fruits and instead of milk with some cereals, especially homemade granola and wheatberry salad.
- If you are lactose intolerant but like the taste of milk and other dairy products, talk to your doctor or pharmacist about using the enzyme lactase—as a food additive or in pill form—which may counteract the bloating effects of milk.
- If you don't like milk or are lactose intolerant, or if you don't eat any animal products, calcium-enriched soy products are a good source for you. Calcium-enriched soy milk is an excellent substitute for dairy milk in most recipes, and it has other nutritionally beneficial properties of its own, such as isoflavones.
- When buying tofu, check the label to be sure it's a type that is made with calcium sulfate, which will provide you with 30 percent of your daily calcium needs; one that is not made with calcium sulfate will provide only 10 percent.

- Firm cheeses such as cheddar, Parmesan, Jack and others are packed with calcium and packed with flavor, too, so that a little goes a long way. One ounce of grated Parmesan can cover quite a large territory on top of a casserole or sprinkled over a green salad.
- Nonfat dry milk is low in calories, very rich in calcium, and it's cholesterol-free. It adds tenderness to breads and biscuits without tampering with the flavor and can be used in many other recipes calling for milk.
- Protein-fortified dairy products—milk, yogurt, and cottage and cream cheeses, including nonfat items—can contain up to and beyond twice as much calcium as ordinary dairy foods.

SUPPLEMENTS ARE NOT A LAST RESORT

In the best of all possible worlds, we would all eat so perfectly that each of us would be in complete nutritional balance . . . unfortunately, this is not a reality. Many of us do get the nutrients our bodies need from the food we eat and, perhaps, from one multivitamin pill a day. For us, most vitamin- or mineral-specific supplements are superfluous, or at best, icing on the cake. But in the case of calcium supplements, there are many people, especially women, whose need for calcium and vitamin D is not being met by food alone, even when augmented by a daily multivitamin pill. For them, supplements may make the difference between a steady loss of bone density and maintaining healthy bones for life. There are a bewildering number of calcium supplements from which to choose. Here are the some of the issues you should consider.

How to decide if you need to take a calcium/vitamin D supplement

1. Estimate how much calcium you get in your daily diet, using the table beginning on page 89.
2. Look at your age category and the DRI on pages 87 and 91.

3. Calculate the difference and make that up either by adding more calcium-rich foods to your diet or by taking supplements.

If you take a supplement, which type should it be?

There are two main formulations of calcium supplements: *calcium citrate* and *calcium carbonate.* Calcium citrate is more easily absorbed than calcium carbonate, but both types have been shown to be effective in improving bone health, when combined with vitamin D.

Rule of thumb: Try calcium citrate first. It can be taken after eating or on an empty stomach. If possible, take your supplement later in the day as calcium is better absorbed when taken without the presence of other food. If you don't tolerate calcium citrate (which most people do), switch to calcium carbonate. Calcium carbonate should be taken with a meal. It can give you gas, and some people become constipated, so take it in small doses.

A third supplement formulation is made up of powdered or crushed materials such as oyster shell, bone meal or dolomite, which are rich in calcium. Use caution in taking these supplements. Some of them are not well absorbed because they don't dissolve easily in the stomach, and some of the sources for the supplements can be contaminated with trace compounds that are toxic.

Be sure that whatever supplement you take contains vitamin D or, if not, that you are receiving vitamin D from another multivitamin supplement.

Do not take more calcium or vitamin D than you need

Supplements are a form of medication—remember that you are also getting these nutrients from foods. Excessive dosages of calcium (more than 1,000 milligrams, or 1 gram, a day from supplementation) or vitamin D (2,000 IU a day from all sources) can be dangerous and can actually reverse the beneficial effects of sufficient amounts of these nutrients.

At the moment, there is no evidence that calcium supplements containing such trace minerals as magnesium, copper, and other nutrients are more effective. Although these minerals may in themselves help promote healthy

Is there lead in calcium supplements?

A recent study in the *Journal of the American Medical Association* (*JAMA*) examined the lead content of a number of over-the-counter calcium supplements. The investigators tested twenty-two calcium supplements and found that eight of the supplements had detectable levels of lead. Lead can cause anemia, hypertension, and brain and kidney damage, and in children it can cause permanent cognitive impairment and problems with behavior. Because of these serious health consequences, laws were enacted in the 1970s to require lead-free gas and paints. Since then there has been an 80% decline in blood lead levels in the United States and a dramatic decrease in lead toxicity, especially in children.

The findings reported in *JAMA* are disturbing because many people rely on calcium supplements—in addition to whole foods—to meet the DRI for calcium. We know that calcium is essential for healthy bones and we assume that our calcium supplement is safe and beneficial to our health. Not all products are equal and the same holds true for calcium supplements. I choose to take Citracal calcium and vitamin D supplements, a brand that does not contain detectable amounts of lead.

bones, they have not been shown to be of any additional help when taken supplementally.

I believe that eating food that promotes strong bones for life promotes overall health and longevity. We should be careful not to fall into an "eat for the disease of the month" syndrome. When I eat well, which is most of the time, I feel great, and I know that I'm helping to strengthen my bones as well as my heart, skin, eyes—in fact my whole body. This is a goal I hope all of us can work toward.

But nutrition is only a piece of the puzzle for achieving and maintaining strong bones. Genetics, sex, race, exercise, and lifestyle are also determinants, as they are for every other aspect of our health, and some of these factors are beyond our control at present.

I am sure that within the next five to ten years, enormous progress will be made in finding ways to reverse or cure osteoporosis, through medications and through better understanding of nutrition. Until then, your understanding of your own nutritional goals and your awareness of what you eat are the best ways to control many aspects of your good health. In terms of strong bones, those goals should include adequate amounts of calcium and vitamin D as well as plenty of exercise, all of which have been shown overwhelmingly to promote good bone health.

CHAPTER 7

Protein

Getting the Right Balance

———————— ❖ ————————

The only time in my life I gained weight (without being pregnant) was when I was in my early twenties. Several of my friends were on a high-protein diet—very popular at that time. I knew nothing about nutrition in those days, so I decided to try it to see if I could lose the weight. Within a day of being on the diet, I was so dizzy and exhausted that I couldn't even walk up a flight of stairs for fear of passing out. All I could do was sit around. Needless to say, I went off the diet very quickly, started eating normally again, and felt better immediately. Since I was very active, the weight came off.

Notoriously popular protein diets have come and gone, and they will keep coming back—as long as anyone is overweight and wants a quick fix. These diets have always been dangerous, but they also help you lose weight fast, and that is why they are popular. But what you really lose is water and lean tissue—and very little fat. You do not solve the problem of what to do when you inevitably start eating a normal, well-balanced diet again, and that's when you regain the weight.

High-protein diets vary from not so dangerous to very dangerous indeed (the diets with extremely limited carbohydrate intake). But one good thing the diets have done is to raise the question of how much protein we need to eat every day, a question that the scientific community has also been rigorously investigating as well.

There is a large gap, however, between the recommendations of the scientific, public-health community and those of the fad diets advocating high-protein regimens.

PROTEIN IN YOUR BODY

Much of your body is made up of protein: your hair, fingernails, muscles, much of your bone, internal organs, skin, eyes, and blood, as well as many compounds within the body, such as hormones and enzymes.

Protein is essential to many life processes. Within the blood, it is important for maintaining blood pressure and water balance inside and outside of the cells. Proteins are required to help transport most substances in and out of the body's cells. For instance, glucose transporters and insulin are both proteins that help bring glucose from the bloodstream into cells.

How the body makes protein

Proteins are extremely complex substances synthesized by the body from amino acids. Amino acids are supplied by protein in the food you eat. When you take in protein, enzymes in the stomach break it down into individual amino acids, which are then absorbed by the small intestines and transported via the bloodstream to the liver and other organs. These amino acids are linked in a vast number of different sequences to make specific proteins in the body.

Amino acids are themselves compounds of carbon, oxygen, and hydrogen (similar to fats and carbohydrates) and nitrogen. The nitrogen of the amino group gives proteins their distinctive characteristics. There are twenty amino acids, and each is unique.

Essential amino acids are the nine amino acids the body cannot manufacture by itself. They must be supplied by the protein in the foods that you eat.

Nonessential amino acids can be supplied by other proteins that you eat or synthesized by the body from other amino acids and fat and carbohydrate fragments already present in the body, without supplementation from ingested protein.

Every day your body requires a specific amount of protein from which it will synthesize new proteins to keep you strong and healthy. Some of this dietary protein must contain the essential amino acids in order for optimal synthesis to occur.

For example, if you ate only wheat products all day, every day, and never ate any other source of protein, your diet would be deficient in lysine, one of the essential amino acids. You would be able to make some proteins using the amino acids in the wheat, but you would not be able to utilize all of them because you would need the lysine to complete the process. In such a case, lysine would be called a *limiting amino acid* because it limits protein synthesis. However, if you ate some beans at the same time as you ate the wheat, the lysine in the beans would complement the protein and synthesis could proceed.

Nitrogen balance

Proteins in the body are constantly in flux. They are being synthesized, put to work, broken down, recycled, repaired—in short, they are always changing. In this state of continuous flux, most of the nitrogen in proteins is usually conserved, but some is inevitably lost in urine and feces.

In order to maintain health, the body needs to be in nitrogen balance, which means that the protein (nitrogen) consumed must equal the protein lost through excretion. Most healthy adults are in *nitrogen balance.*

Growing infants, children, and pregnant women, who need protein for the formation of bones, muscle, and other tissue, take in more nitrogen than they lose and are said to be in *positive nitrogen balance.*

Starvation, anorexia, or other severe illness or distress such as injury, fever, and infection may force the body to use protein as fuel and put the body into *negative nitrogen balance.* When this occurs, the body loses important lean tissue, especially muscle.

In well-nourished, healthy individuals, when too much dietary protein is taken in and not used, it is degraded, used as energy, or stored as body fat.

Roles that protein plays in your body

Your body contains tens of thousands of different kinds of protein, each with a specific purpose, which is determined by a complex biochemical process within each cell during protein synthesis.

Versatility is the best way to describe protein's activity in your body. Protein is needed to give structure to collagen in connective tissue, muscles, hair, bone and teeth, ligaments, tendons, skin, and other organs. Enzymes are also proteins. Enzymes build and transform substances, and they facilitate the transformation of one substance into another. Proteins act as hormones by regulating body processes and as antibodies to defend against disease. Proteins participate in regulating fluid and electrolyte balance as well as regulating acid-base balance and transporting nutrients throughout the body.

Protein as an energy source

Typically, very little protein is used as energy. When necessary, that is, when glucose and fatty acids are in short supply, the body is forced to use protein as an energy source in the form of glucose. This conversion is accomplished when the body removes nitrogen from amino acids, leaving a carbon structure that can be used as energy. Excess protein in the diet, an insufficient intake of carbohydrate, high-intensity exercise, and fever or other sickness can all trigger the conversion to greater use of protein for energy.

PROTEIN IN FOODS

There are numerous dietary sources of protein, but with considerable differences in the amounts and the quality of protein they contain.

Complete proteins

A complete protein supplies all the essential amino acids (the ones the body cannot manufacture on its own) in the right amounts for the body to synthesize its own protein efficiently. Complete proteins contain varying amounts of nonessential amino acids as well. The highest-quality proteins are derived from animals: eggs, milk and milk products such as cheese and yogurt, meats, including beef, lamb, pork, chicken and fish. Animal-derived proteins also contain significant amounts of iron, zinc, and B vitamins, with meats also supplying omega-6 fatty acid.

The only complete protein derived from plants is in soy and soy food products.

Incomplete proteins

Incomplete proteins lack at least one of the essential amino acids or do not contain sufficient amounts of them to permit the body to make its own protein. Incomplete proteins are those from plants: legumes, many nuts and seeds as well as nut butters (hummus, peanut or cashew butter), a few vegetables, and grains, including wheat, rice, corn, and others.

Complementary proteins

A complementary protein is the combination of two or more incomplete proteins that together provide enough of the essential amino acids in the correct amounts for efficient use by the body. These combinations, eaten over the course of a day, usually provide all the complete proteins you need for optimal nutrition, if you eat a variety of foods and take in sufficient energy.

A typical complementary protein is a grain combined with a legume: rice and beans in any one of hundreds of ethnic variations; a grain and tofu and broccoli; peanut butter and whole-grain bread. Information about vegetarian diets is given in greater detail in Chapter 8.

A little goes a long way
Vegetable proteins can be greatly improved in quality by the addition of even a small amount of animal protein. For instance, adding cheese to a bean and rice burrito transforms a complementary protein (the grains and legume combo) into a high-quality, complete protein.

HOW MUCH PROTEIN DO YOU NEED?

The amount of protein needed for a healthy, well-balanced diet is a hotly debated subject in the scientific community, and in the fad diet community and the media as well. It's interesting to note the vast divergence among these sectors. While the scientists are negotiating amounts of protein that differ as much (or as little) as tenths of a gram a day, some of the fad diets tell us that protein should be 30 percent of our calorie intake—twice the amount recommended by the RDAs (Recommended Daily Allowances). Some fad diets are even recommending that 50 percent of your calories be protein! Who is right?

A range of recommendations

There is a wide range of recommendations for protein. To give you an idea of the different approaches to this very serious issue, here are three recommendations for diet composition representing three separate viewpoints. The first of these diets is the one supported by scientific research and the one that I recommend as well.

Majority of national scientific organizations, including the National Academy of Sciences
   10 to 15 percent of calories from protein (50 to 80 grams for women)
   55 to 60 percent of calories from carbohydrates (rich in fruits, vegetables, and whole grains)
   No more than 30 percent from fat

A more aggressive approach
   30 percent of calories from protein
   40 percent from carbohydrates
   30 percent from fat

While there is no scientific support for this amount of protein in the diet, it probably is not dangerous. It is, however, a hard diet to follow because when protein intake is so high, it's difficult to hold the fat to only 30 percent of calories. It is also difficult to get enough fruits and vegetables on this type of diet, so optimal vitamin and mineral intake may be compromised.

High-protein advocates
40 to 50 percent of calories from protein
10 to 20 percent from carbohydrates
40 percent from fat

This diet is downright dangerous, as I will discuss later. There is no scientific evidence that this diet is healthy, and in fact there is information that it is *not* healthy and can result in loss of lean tissue and bone, heart problems, kidney problems, and other deleterious effects. It does lead to short-term weight loss, but to the detriment of overall health.

Protein Content of Typical Foods

FOOD	AMOUNT	PROTEIN (GRAMS)	CALORIES
EGG	1 medium	6	74
DAIRY			
Milk 2%	8 oz	8	121
Cheddar cheese	1 oz	7	113
Camembert	1 oz	6	84
Ice cream	½ cup	2.5	133
MEAT (COOKED—LEAN)			
Beef	4 oz	32	311
Chicken/turkey	1 oz	34	177
Fish	4 oz	30	158
Lamb	1 oz	29	292
Pork	1 oz	25	201

(continued)

LEGUMES (COOKED)			
Soybeans	½ cup	14	149
Edamame	½ cup	11	127
Tofu (firm)	½ cup	20	183
Soy milk	8 oz	7	80
Other beans	½ cup	8	114
Peas	½ cup	4	62
Peanuts	¼ cup	10	209
Peanut butter	2 T	8	190
GRAINS			
Bread	1 slice	3	65
Bagel (3.5-inch)	1	7	195
Rice	½ cup	2	102
Bulgur		3	75
Pasta	½ cup	4	98
Flour	1 cup	13	455
Oatmeal cereal (hot)	½ cup	3	73
Cold cereal	½ cup	1–3 (varies)	50 (varies)
NUTS			
General	¼ cup	6	209
Seeds			
Sesame	1 T	2	47
Sunflower	1 T	6	160
VEGETABLES			
General	½ cup	1–3	Varies
Potatoes	1 medium	5	220
FRUITS			
General	½ cup	< 2	Varies

How do I know if I'm getting enough protein?

Most healthy adults do get enough protein if they eat a varied diet that includes all the food groups in sensible proportions. Even if you don't eat meat per se, but you do eat eggs and dairy, you are very likely getting enough protein. Look at the table beginning on page 105 and calculate how much protein you get on average each day.

This worksheet will help you check whether you are getting enough protein to meet your requirements. Remember to include foods eaten at meals and for snacks. Keep in mind that serving sizes can differ, and what you see on your plate may be more, or less, than the serving sizes on the chart.

LIST FOODS BELOW	SERVING SIZE	APPROXIMATE AMOUNT OF PROTEIN
ADD UP ALL PROTEIN-RICH FOODS	TOTAL:	

The recommended amount of protein is 50 to 80 grams per day. If you are active, keep your protein intake closer to 80 grams a day.

People at risk for protein deficiency

While it is easy for most people to get enough protein, I am continually amazed at the number of people who restrict their diets in one way or another and consequently may get insufficient protein.

People with restricted fat intake or eating disorders
Deficiency is a risk for those who severely limit their intake of fat. Because proteins are usually present in foods that also contain some fat, people who attempt to eliminate most fats from their diets may get insufficient protein. People with eating disorders usually restrict their intake of energy, or they purge themselves after a meal. These people are particularly at risk for protein deficiency.

Athletes
The first study I ever conducted at Tufts, in the early 1980s, was with young women athletes, who either maintained their menstrual cycles while they were training or did not. The women who did not maintain their menstrual cycles also had disordered eating patterns, and over 50 percent of them were not even meeting the recommended amount of protein despite the fact that they were all athletes and should have known better! We believe that the pattern of disordered eating, and especially the low protein intake, contributed greatly to the development of amenorrhea (lack of a menstrual cycle).

Pregnancy and lactation
During pregnancy and lactation, the body should be producing more protein: in pregnancy, to grow the fetus; in lactation, to produce high-quality milk. During these periods in your life, in order to stay well nourished, you should eat a little more protein so that you don't borrow from your own protein stores. The Recommended Daily Allowance for protein for pregnant and lactating women is no less than 60 to 65 grams.

Elderly
Another group particularly at risk for low protein intake are the elderly, primarily older women who have a low calorie intake to begin with. About 25

percent of elderly women are not meeting the RDA for protein. Marginal protein intake can contribute to frailty and sickness in the elderly.

Strict vegetarians (vegans)
Vegans can also eat insufficient high-quality protein unless they plan their meals carefully.

The poor
The poor in the United States and especially in developing countries are especially vulnerable to low protein intakes and malnutrition because high-quality proteins (meats, dairy, and eggs) are much more expensive than carbohydrates or even fat.

OVERCONSUMPTION: THE DANGERS OF HIGH-PROTEIN DIETS

High-protein, low-carbohydrate diets are risky for your health. Although doctors who promote these diets tell you otherwise, don't believe them.

The high costs of high-protein diets

The longer you are on a high-protein, low-carbohydrate diet, the more deleterious the effects on your body.

- *Heart disease.* In order to get as much protein as a high-protein diet recommends, you must eat large amounts of animal protein, which carries with it large quantities of animal (saturated) fat and cholesterol. This combination has been linked repeatedly with higher rates of heart disease.
- *Cancer.* Population studies have also shown a correlation between high intakes of animal protein and cancer of the colon, breast, kidneys, pancreas, and prostate.
- *Bone loss.* As protein consumption increases well over the recommended amount, calcium excretion rises, which can contribute to

bone loss. Women who consume large amounts of animal proteins should pay close attention to their calcium intake.

- *Insufficient fiber and nutrients.* Restricted intake of whole grains, fruits, and vegetables deprives the body of the nutrients and phytochemicals that protect against disease. Although supplementation is recommended in these diet plans, it rarely delivers the health benefits you would get from real food.
- *Loss of appetite.* The monotony of a high-protein diet eventually can result in a lack of interest in eating, or loss of appetite, and to eating less food overall, which can result in a lower energy intake and extreme fatigue.
- *Difficulty losing more weight.* Long-term low calorie consumption seriously depresses the metabolic rate, making it harder and harder to lose weight—almost as if your body were willfully resisting your desire to weaken it further.

The wasting process

The brain and red blood cells use glucose as their chief source of energy. When carbohydrate intake is limited or virtually nil, the body turns to its own protein tissues such as muscles and the liver, breaks down those tissues into amino acids, and then uses the amino acids to make glucose. The syndrome of body protein tissue breakdown is called the wasting process.

Ketosis

One of the most potentially serious effects of a high-protein, low-carbohydrate diet is ketosis, which occurs when the brain is no longer getting enough glucose for fuel. At that point the body turns to its store of fats to provide an alternate energy source, called ketone bodies. While ketone bodies can be used as fuel by the brain, they are an inferior source of energy, and they are toxic. In order to dispose of them, the body flushes them out in urine, which accounts for the rapid and extreme weight loss people experience after just a few days on high-protein diets.

Some of the adverse effects of a low-carbohydrate, ketogenic diet are:

- Dizziness
- Low blood pressure
- Fatigue
- Nausea
- Dehydration
- Constipation
- Foul taste in mouth
- Foul breath

I experienced several of these very unpleasant side effects myself many years ago when I went on a high-protein, low-carbohydrate diet. Some people can adapt to a ketogenic diet over time, but they will continue to experience these side effects. The harmful results are that they also continue to lose water, muscle, and bone rapidly while losing only modest amounts of fat tissue. At a certain point the water loss slows down, and weight loss slows dramatically, but the body is still losing muscle and other lean tissue and some fat.

High-protein, low-carbohydrate diets are also very taxing on the heart. When you lose electrolytes and become dehydrated, your heart must work harder to pump blood. People have been known to die from these diets.

Protein requirements for athletes

Our laboratory at Tufts University has been among the leaders in investigating protein requirements, conducting several seminal studies over the last 20 years. The studies have ranged from endurance athletes to older men and women. All of the studies have shown that protein requirements of healthy, active adults are between the RDA of 0.8 g/kg body weight and 1.4 g/kg body weight. Even at twice the RDA, or 1.6 g/kg body weight, this comes to 58 to 66 grams of protein a day, or about 13 percent of calories in a 2,000-calorie-per-day diet—well within the recommended amounts of protein.

Studies in other laboratories around the country have shown that elite athletes or those just starting a rigorous training program may have slightly higher requirements, but these increased requirements still amount to no more than 15 percent of calories coming from protein. In addition, the more a person exercises, the more calories she will need to maintain body weight. In a high-quality diet, with a variety of foods, protein intake will also rise as calories increase, as will all the other nutrients, and the athlete will be able to meet her requirements easily.

There is absolutely no scientific evidence that eating a diet with higher than 15 percent protein, or 80 grams in a 2,200-calorie-a-day diet, has any added benefit for health or exercise performance.

Research does show that the only people who need more protein when exercising are body builders trying to get "ripped." Such athletes are usually on a relatively low-calorie diet and are working out a lot. In order to protect the body from muscle loss, an intake of 30 percent or more of calories is recommended. Although this is an extreme example, it does show that protein requirements go up as energy intake goes down.

Amino acid/protein supplements

Although they are sold in health food stores, through magazines, and in other venues, protein supplements are unnecessary for healthy, well-nourished adults. Claims about their potential benefits—that they help athletes build muscle, dieters lose weight, women strengthen their fingernails, improve sleep, relieve pain or depression, and more—are wholly unfounded.

STRATEGIES FOR MANAGING
YOUR PROTEIN INTAKE

Awareness of what you eat and delight in eating are the keys to managing all your nutritional needs. Here are a few tips on getting the right amount of protein every day:

- When you look down at your plate at every meal, some of the foods you see should contain significant amounts of protein. For example, at lunch or dinner, you should be looking at rice and broccoli, *and* some beans or fish or a small amount of animal protein to extend the complementary proteins of grain, legumes, and vegetable.
- Eat protein from a variety of sources, not just animal protein.
- Complementary proteins are among the most satisfying food combinations in many ethnic cuisines, particularly grains and legumes eaten together.
- Soy food products, such as soy milk, tofu, edamame, and soy flour, are nutritionally versatile; they can add protein to a strictly vegetarian diet and be used by themselves or incorporated into other dishes. See Chapter 8 for more about the health benefits of soy foods.
- Dairy foods are an important source of protein as well as calcium and vitamin D.
- Fish is so healthy, and it's crammed with protein. New research has shown that people who eat fish on average at least once a week have about a 50 percent reduction in cardiac death. This is most likely due to the high amount of health-promoting omega-3 fatty acids contained in fish (see Chapter 9).

For the lay public, there are few more controversial nutritional topics than how much protein is required for optimal health. Despite the confusion and the conflicting information, study after study has shown that where all else is equal, where the rest of the foods we eat are high-quality and unprocessed, we need no more than 15 percent protein for optimal health.

This goal is easily met by eating a variety of foods, some of which contain protein. Nothing tastes better to me than that.

Eggs are the perfect protein

You might even call eggs the mother of all proteins, because they are the standard against which all proteins are compared. Despite this, for years the public health community has told us we must limit our consumption of eggs because they are high in cholesterol. Some people even eat egg substitutes to minimize cholesterol. It's sad.

Fortunately the scientists are taking another look at eggs, and we're discovering some interesting new facts. A recent Harvard study showed that eating as much as one egg a day (or seven eggs in the course of one week) did not increase vascular disease at all. It's great news because eggs are packed with important nutrients. Egg yolks are one of the few foods that contain vitamin D, and they also have some vitamin B_{12}, riboflavin, and folate. One egg gives you about 75 calories and a significant amount of your daily protein.

And there's more. There are now omega-3-enriched eggs, which are produced by feeding laying hens a special diet containing 10 to 20 percent ground flaxseed. Since flaxseed is higher in omega-3 fatty acids and lower in saturated fatty acids than other grains, the eggs produced by these hens are higher in omega-3 fatty acids, but not in overall fat or cholesterol. The eggs, packed in cartons and marked as omega-3 enriched, are sold in many local supermarkets.

CHAPTER 8

Vegetarianism and Soy

A Perfect Partnership

❖

When I was in college, I did what at least half of my friends were doing—I became a vegetarian. It was as much a decision about social issues as it was about health. With no previous kitchen experience at all, and without a clue about what I was doing, I enthusiastically began to cook a great many vegetarian meals. My two roommates called my meals mystery food, and they were right.

But an important change occurred as part of my new diet—I started to eat more soy foods and found that I enjoyed them. This was back in the late 1970s and early '80s, when it was difficult to find even tofu in food stores, to say nothing of other soy products. We've come a long way since then.

Vegetarianism is no longer just a social issue, it is a health issue. Not only are there a lot more choices among soy foods, we now have many more options for healthy, tasty vegetarian diets. The availability of these foods and the growing interest in vegetarianism has in turn spurred the publication of new vegetarian cookbooks, from the most basic to the most sophisticated, giving all of us the ability to make delicious meals.

While I do eat some meat now, the majority of my meals are vegetarian.

Since having children, we eat a lot more soy foods—my kids were introduced to them at an early age and love them. I make it a point to eat soy several times a week because I like it and because I know that it helps promote and maintain our family's good health.

We are learning more about the health benefits of a diet that is low in meat and high in vegetable protein. At the same time, we are learning more about the health benefits of soy foods. The combination of low meat intake and soy foods is a perfect partnership for good health—especially for women.

VEGETARIAN BASICS

There are several forms of vegetarianism. They run the gamut from a diet that excludes red meat, fish, and poultry but does include dairy products and eggs to a diet with no animal-based foods at all. The motivations for becoming a vegetarian are as varied as the diets themselves: dislike of animal foods, health concerns, and political or religious beliefs, among others. Whatever the impetus, you can have a healthy, nutritionally sound vegetarian diet—particularly with help from soy foods.

Here are four common types of vegetarians:

- *Semi-vegetarians,* who typically exclude red meat but occasionally eat some fish or poultry.
- *Lacto-ovo-vegetarians,* whose diet includes milk and milk products and eggs but no meat, poultry, or fish.
- *Lacto-vegetarians,* who eat milk and milk products but exclude meat, poultry, fish, and eggs.
- *Vegans,* who eat only plant-based foods and exclude meat, poultry, fish, eggs, and dairy products.

What is the case for a vegetarian diet?

For several decades, scientists have been examining the effects of a vegetarian diet and the risk of a number of different chronic diseases on longevity. These investigations have demonstrated the benefits of diets very low in meat or altogether meatless. The benefits include decreased risk of coronary artery disease (CAD), high blood pressure, obesity, and cancer.

On the face of it, it would seem that if you are currently a vegetarian, you may enjoy a longer, healthier life at least in part because of what you eat—or don't eat. But food is only part of the equation. Many vegetarians are also health-conscious. For that reason, they don't smoke or overindulge in alcohol, and they lead active lives. So while the vegetarian diet itself may be health-promoting, as some of the studies indicate, accompanying lifestyle factors may be equally important.

On the other hand, if you eat meat, poultry, fish, or dairy products, I am not suggesting that you give them up. The research, as you will see, is not sufficiently definitive for you to banish nutrient-rich foods that you enjoy.

What I do suggest is that you try to develop some of the same awareness of healthy eating and a healthy lifestyle that so many vegetarians have. Start getting your protein from a variety of sources that includes beans, fish, soy, eggs, poultry, and only limited amounts of meat. If you are sedentary, begin regular exercise, and stop smoking, if that is your habit now.

What the research shows

As early as 1982, a study of over 10,000 people, published in the *American Journal of Clinical Nutrition* showed a significantly decreased risk of heart disease in vegetarians, particularly among men.

Later studies have revealed reductions of cancer and heart-disease-related deaths among vegetarians, as well as lower blood pressure and lower LDL cholesterol. In 1994, a British study found a 20 percent decrease in total mortality in people who ate no meat.

This does sound like a strong argument for becoming a vegetarian, but it's really only half the picture. Important research has shown that fish containing omega-3 and omega-6 fatty acids also have health-promoting properties. Clearly, eggs and dairy foods have a special place in a healthy diet—eggs because they are an excellent source of protein and vitamin A, and dairy products because they are among the best, if not the absolute best, sources of calcium and vitamin D. Even beef, which is packed with minerals such as iron and zinc, can have a place in a healthy diet. The basic problem for a lot of people who eat meat is that they eat too much of it too often.

The Vegetarian Food Guide Pyramid (VFGP)

If you are already a vegetarian or thinking about becoming one, the VFGP is an excellent tool to help you meet all of your nutritional needs without eat-

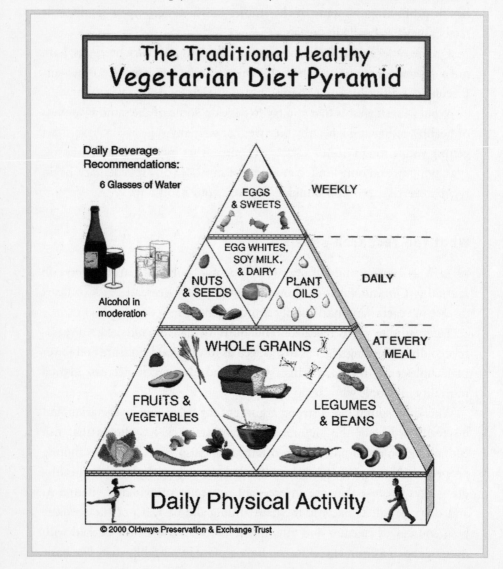

The Traditional Healthy
Vegetarian Diet Pyramid

Daily Beverage Recommendations:

6 Glasses of Water

Alcohol in moderation

EGGS & SWEETS — WEEKLY

EGG WHITES, SOY MILK, & DAIRY

NUTS & SEEDS

PLANT OILS — DAILY

WHOLE GRAINS — AT EVERY MEAL

FRUITS & VEGETABLES

LEGUMES & BEANS

Daily Physical Activity

© 2000 Oldways Preservation & Exchange Trust

ing meat. Traditionally, most vegetarians eat eggs and dairy products, and that is the basis for this pyramid.

Awareness, planning, and eating a variety of complementary foods—especially nuts, legumes, seeds, and soy—every day are essential to meet your dietary needs, especially if you are a vegan. I believe that you can eat very well as a vegetarian, or you can eat poorly. The key is making sure you get all the energy and nutrients you need through a variety of nutrient-rich foods.

Vegans may have more difficulty meeting their requirements for the nutrients that are found in abundance in meat and dairy products, such as calcium, vitamin D, vitamin B_{12}, magnesium, zinc, and iron. If you are a vegan, it may be prudent to take a multi-vitamin-mineral supplement to prevent deficiencies.

Parents of vegan children should pay particular attention to the special needs children have for calcium, vitamin D, and protein.

HOW SOY CAN REDUCE
THE RISK OF CHRONIC DISEASE

The health benefits of the many food products derived from soybeans have been recognized for millennia in Asia. In the United States, people interested in natural whole foods, alternative health, and Asian culture have long touted soybeans as the food of the future, especially tofu in its various incarnations. It is only in the last two decades that the health-promoting value of soybeans has been seriously studied by the Western medical establishment.

Preliminary research

The First International Symposium on the Role of Soy in Preventing and Treating Chronic Disease was held in February 1994. At that time, there were so few scientists studying soy that each of them knew all of the relevant research—it was so limited. The Second International Symposium was held 1996 and the Third in November 1999. Although little was published about isoflavones in soy before 1993, over 1,000 studies were published between 1994 and 1999!

The history of soy

Soybeans are a legume that have been grown for more than 5,000 years in China, their cultivation first recorded in about 2800 B.C. The beans spread to Japan and Korea around A.D. 600, reached Europe in the 1600s, and arrived in America in the mid–eighteenth century.

Soybean cultivation here began in earnest in the mid-1920s, but soybeans didn't become an important food crop in Western cultures until after World War II. By then, the cotton crop in the South basically had destroyed the soil and depleted it of nitrogen. Farmers knew that legumes would help to "fix" nitrogen back into the soil, so they started growing soybeans. The vast majority of soybeans are now grown in the Western hemisphere, with 75 percent produced in the United States, where they are now a major export crop.

I find soy foods interesting because they are a good basic food, but they also seem to have medicinal qualities that make them almost a functional food. (See page 76 for more about functional foods.) From about 1950 to 1990, soy foods were recommended by the health food community because of their high-quality protein. This is no longer the main reason for the interest in and promotion of soy foods; the isoflavones are, and it is their potential to reduce the risk of numerous chronic diseases that has engaged the attention and resources of the scientific community, not to mention the food producers.

Recent epidemiological research demonstrates that populations whose diets are rich in soy foods have reduced rates of heart disease and breast, lung, colon, and prostate cancer. These populations also experience fewer menopausal problems and have improved bone health.

Nutrient-packed soybeans

The early proponents of soybeans were right: They are equivalent to animal protein in terms of protein quality. They have the highest protein content of any plant-based food, and, most importantly, the protein is complete, meaning that all of the essential amino acids are in the right complement, making soybeans a high-quality protein. They also contain a significant amount of fat, but the fat is unsaturated and high in omega-3 fatty acids, the kind of fat that is beneficial and helps reduce the risk of heart disease.

Soybeans (and all legumes) are an important source of carbohydrates, B vitamins (including folate), vitamin K, zinc, potassium, magnesium, calcium, iron, and fiber.

Henry Ford—a man ahead of his time

Henry Ford, the automotive genius, was an innovator in the realm of agriculture as well. In 1931, he sponsored studies into the industrial and nutritional potential of soybeans.

It was Ford's conviction that soy was an ideal human food (it was already widely used as animal feed). He had his personal chef develop soy recipes, and, during the 1934 Chicago World's Fair, he threw a dinner party for thirty people at which all sixteen courses included soy in one form or another. His favorite soybean cookie recipe, which includes soy margarine, soy milk, soybean flour, roasted soybean nuts, and four cups of chocolate chips (the recipe makes 120 cookies), can be found on a number of soy websites.

Ford's interest in putting agricultural products to industrial use was visionary and far-reaching. Although soy was one of his primary interests (he was photographed in 1935 wearing a suit made of soybeans), other plants were not neglected. In 1941 Ford presented his "biological" car. Seventy percent of the body was made from an assortment of fibers ranging from hemp to field straw, and the remaining 30 percent from a filler of soybean and a liquid bioresin. Other parts of the car, including pedals, door handles, and gearshift knobs, also originated in soybeans. In a famous photo, Ford is shown wielding an ax against the trunk, but to no avail: the car remained undamaged.

Phytoestrogens

Soybeans also are a source of phytoestrogens, the hormone-like versions of phytochemicals, which may be responsible for much of the health-promoting qualities of soy. In soybeans, isoflavones are the phytoestrogens that have been identified as beneficial to health. The two most abundant isoflavones in soy are genistein and daidzein.

Phytoestrogens and cancer prevention

Phytoestrogens act as weak estrogens. Genistein and other isoflavones function protectively by competing with the more potent estrogens within the body for available binding sites on estrogen receptors on the surfaces of cells. This dilution effectively decreases the amount of potent estrogens that can bind to the receptors and sometimes promote cancer, and this decrease can lead to a lower risk of breast cancer. Yet the isoflavones still act as estrogens, albeit weak ones, and provide enough estrogen to diminish hot flashes and improve bone health.

Genistein also inhibits the action of a variety of key enzymes involved in the cancer process. In a third mechanism, genistein inhibits the formation of the new blood vessels needed for the growth and spread of tumors.

Phytoestrogens help reduce cholesterol

Dozens of controlled clinical studies have shown that the phytoestrogens in soy protein also exert positive effects in lowering the risk of heart disease by helping to transport LDL cholesterol to the liver, where it can be broken down and destroyed.

For this reason, soy products are now among the select group of foods for which the FDA allows a health claim. As of October 1999, the FDA approved the following statement, which can appear on any food containing at least 6.25 grams of soy protein: "25 grams of soy protein a day as part of a diet low in saturated fat and cholesterol, may reduce the risk of heart disease." To take in this much soy protein and achieve the cholesterol-lowering effect, two to three servings of soy every day are required (see table on page 129).

Decrease menopausal symptoms

A diet rich in soy products may also help reduce the symptoms of meno-
pause. In an eighteen-week study conducted by Bowman Gray School of
Medicine in North Carolina, women taking 20 grams of powdered soy protein added to their breakfasts experienced fewer severe menopausal symptoms, such as hot flashes and night sweats. As an added benefit, their total
cholesterol levels dropped an average of 10 percent.

A tale of two cultures

In 1994, in a review of the literature done by a scientist at McGill University
in Montreal, a cross-cultural study comparing menopausal Japanese women
to menopausal American and Canadian women was published. It showed
that:

- The Japanese group had the highest consumption of soy, with a
  daily intake of 200 mgs of isoflavones, while the American and
  Canadian intake was less than 5 mgs a day.
- Post-menopausal Japanese women rarely reported having perimen-
  opausal symptoms, which were common among Western women.
- Post-menopausal Japanese women had lower rates of osteoporosis
  and heart disease, and they had a longer life expectancy.

Soy futures

Research is currently underway to follow up on studies that have already
shown a link between consumption of soy foods and a lowered risk of such
diseases as prostate cancer, colon cancer, and osteoporosis. I firmly believe
that, as more studies are completed and more facts are known about the
health-promoting qualities of soybeans, the time will come when soy products are automatically included in the diets of a vast majority of Americans.
That's when the future will be here.

SOY FOODS

There are over 1,000 varieties of soybeans, but only a few are grown in the United States. Of the more than twenty soy foods produced in this country, many are available now in supermarkets and the rest at health food stores. Here are some of them:

Fresh soybeans (edamame) are harvested while the beans are still green. They are absolutely my favorite type of soy food! They look like baby lima beans, but have a sweeter, nuttier flavor and a less starchy texture. Edamame eaten directly out of the pod, either hot or cold, are the perfect snack food, and I would eat them every day, if we didn't run out of them so quickly at our house.

Shelled edamame are delicious in salads and risottos and mixed with

Did you know . . . ?

- Soybeans are the second largest cash crop in the United States after wheat.
- Half the soybeans grown in this country are exported.
- April is National Soyfoods Month.
- Aside from the soybeans grown for export and those used for food products, the beans are also are used for a staggering number of other nonfood products. According to a list published on the Indiana Soybean Board's website, these include body care products, candles, cleaners, composite materials, crayons, diesel additives, fabric conditioner, flooring, hair conditioners, hair styling aids, hand cleaners, paint removers, pens, polish, shampoos, solvents, waxes for tables and other furniture.
- Recently, soy milk outsold Coca-Cola in Hong Kong.
- Brewed soybeans were used as a coffee substitute during the Civil War.

other vegetables (see recipes). They are available in health-food stores and many supermarkets, parboiled and frozen, still in the pod or shelled, and they require only a few moments of cooking in salted water. If you have a kitchen garden, you might want to plant your own edamame. They are as easy to grow as green beans, and recently I've begun to see fresh edamame at local farmers' markets.

Whole dried soybeans are a good source of protein and fiber, although somewhat bland in flavor. They must be soaked before cooking and can be used in stews and soups.

Soynuts are soaked dried soybeans that have been roasted until brown. They make a delicious, if somewhat caloric, snack. Soynuts are available in health food stores plain and flavored in many ways.

Tofu, or *soybean curd,* is a soft, cheeselike cake made from curdled soybean milk. Tofu comes in a variety of flavors and different degrees of firmness.

Silken tofu is creamy in texture and can be used for dressings, dips, shakes, smoothies, and sauces, and in baked dishes, such as cakes and custards, where you want a smooth texture.

Soft tofu has many of the characteristics of silken tofu, but is a little firmer and more crumbly. Use in salads and in scrambled eggs as well as in baked goods.

Firm, or *regular,* tofu is excellent in stir-fried, grilled, and sautéed dishes, and is also widely used for casseroles, soups, and sandwiches. It is highest of all the forms of tofu in protein, calcium, and fat.

Soybean oil, the oil extracted from whole soybeans, is the most widely used oil in the United States, usually sold as "vegetable oil." It contains no cholesterol and is high in polyunsaturated fat.

Soy flour, made from finely ground roasted soybeans, is higher in protein and lower in carbohydrates than wheat flour. Available in health-food stores, it comes in three varieties: *natural,* or full-fat, which has all the natural soybean oil; *defatted,* with all the fat removed; and *lecithinated,* to which lecithin has been added. The defatted soy flour has a greater concentration of protein. Because soy flour contains no gluten, it is always used in combination with other flours for baking.

Soy milk is a nondairy beverage made from crushed, cooked soybeans. Be sure to buy soy milk fortified with calcium and vitamin D. It can be drunk on its own and used in recipes exactly as dairy milk is: in sauces, soups, baking,

Isoflavone supplements: When skepticism is your best bet

Much of the research into the health-promoting qualities of soy has been done using whole soy foods, such as soy milk, tofu, soy nuts, soy protein added to foods, miso, and others described on these pages.

Most scientists in the field are concerned about the untested effects, especially the estrogenic effects, of isolated isoflavones from soy (whether natural or synthetic) that are sold over the counter in pill and powder form. There is a strong possibility that these supplements may be more harmful than helpful, and until they have been thoroughly tested, I recommend that you stick with whole soy foods and don't experiment with isolated isoflavones or other soy supplements. Whole soy foods also contain other phytochemicals which most likely also have health-promoting qualities.

The average intake of soy isoflavones among Japanese women— *all of it from food, not from supplements*—is 50 to 200 milligrams a day. The effects of an exceedingly high intake of isoflavones—some capsules contain up to 500 milligrams—are still unknown and may be potentially dangerous.

While current research is now also focusing on isolated isoflavones, the long-term health benefits or risk for harmful side effects are still not known. The keys to a healthy diet are moderation in consumption of any one food and eating a wide range of whole foods.

custards, and flavored beverages. Vanilla and chocolate soy milk are also widely available, with the chocolate milk coming in at 50 calories more per eight-ounce cup serving than plain soy milk.

Soy cheese and *soy yogurt* are made from soy milk. Available in a variety of flavors in health-food stores, both the cheese and the yogurt have a creamy texture and are used much the way cream cheese and dairy sour cream are.

Textured soy protein (TSP) is soy flour that is high in protein and often sold in health-food stores as an extender or replacement for meat or poultry. Veggie burgers and sausages are usually made with TSP.

Soy sauce, made from fermented soybeans, originated over 2,500 years ago in China and was first used as a preservative and then as a condiment. *Shoyu* (made with wheat) and *tamari* (generally made without wheat) are the two variants of the sauce that are available widely in supermarkets. They contain no protein and can be high in sodium. Read the bottle label carefully to see that the sauce contains no caramel or corn syrup.

Miso, a fermented soybean paste similar in consistency to peanut butter, is a common flavoring in Japanese cooking. Most of us are familiar with the miso soups found in Japanese restaurants, but miso is also used as a condiment in dips, sauces, dressings, and marinades. Depending on the amount used, it can provide protein, calcium, and some B vitamins. Miso tends to be high in sodium, but there are low-salt varieties available. You can buy it in health food stores. Refrigerate after opening.

Tempeh is a chewy cake made from soybeans mixed with rice, millet, or other grain and then fermented. Tempeh, which is available at health food stores, can be marinated and grilled and used in soups, stews, and spaghetti dishes. It is a good source for protein, but has less calcium.

Genetic engineering

Soybeans, like every other commercial crop grown in the United States, have been subject to a considerable degree of genetic engineering, which has drawn controversy countered by sharp rebukes from industrial giants in the field of seed production. Since 1996 there are more than 4 million acres of farmland that grow genetically engineered (GE) foods.

Soybeans were among the first crops to undergo genetic engineering. Currently it is estimated that more than half of the soy crop is genetically engineered. At first it was done to give the plants better tolerance for herbicides and protection from insects. Now energetic research is going into engineering a soybean with more protein, improved oil content, and more isoflavones.

While this is potentially a worthy endeavor, we still don't know the long-term effects—beneficial or negative—over the next fifty years or so on human health or the health of the environment. For more about genetic engineering and related topics, see Chapter 11.

INCREASE SOY IN YOUR DIET

First, if you have never had soy or it has been a long time since you've tried it, find a good recipe (there are several in this book) and start to experiment. Begin by eating at least two servings of soy every week to get yourself into the habit. Be sure to try edamame, and if you like them, keep a bag in the freezer. They are so delicious you may find that you're eating them more than twice a week.

If you are serious about working toward reducing your risk of heart disease, cancer, osteoporosis, or menopausal symptoms, you will be motivated to work toward eating at least one or two servings of soy per day. This may seem difficult at first, but if you experiment with soy foods, you will soon find a few soy staples—soy milk and edamame, for instance—that you enjoy and that you can use alone or with other foods. Keep those foods on hand.

In my family, we have soy about four times per week. We eat tofu and edamame. My children and husband like soy milk, but I'm not a fan. So I stick with the first two items. Occasionally we have soynuts, and in the winter my husband makes a wonderful miso soup.

Serving sizes

The table below shows the portion sizes and a few nutrient values for a number of soy foods.

SOY FOOD	AMOUNT	CALORIES	PROTEIN g	FAT g
Tofu, firm	½ cup	154	17	9
Tofu, regular	½ cup	76	8	5
Soy milk	8 oz	81	7	5
Edamame	½ cup	127	11	6
Soynuts	¼ cup	203	15	11
Tempeh	½ cup	166	16	6
TSP (textured soy protein)	¼ cup	93	21	1
Miso	1 T	35	2	1
Soy burgers	1 patty (3 oz cooked)	95	14	3
Soy flour, full fat	½ cup	183	15	9

Note: All numbers have been rounded to the nearest whole number. This table shows typical nutritional values for these foods, but values will vary depending on the brand, so check the nutrition facts label.

I am no longer a vegetarian, but I don't eat a lot of meat. I do eat more good-tasting soy foods each week, and my family enjoys them. The fact that soy foods are nutritious—high in protein, omega-3 fatty acids, fiber, and health-promoting isoflavones—makes them a natural for inclusion in a well-rounded, wholesome diet. I have no doubt that we will be reading about the health-promoting qualities of vegetarianism and soy for years to come.

CHAPTER 9

Fats, Sugar, and Salt

The Good, the Bad, and the Ugly

❖

Wow! Talk about an explosive topic: fats, sugar, and salt! Three foods that add so much flavor and pleasure to our diet, three foods that are often the designated culprits—and too often, the scapegoats—in the incidence of obesity, heart disease, diabetes, cancer, and hypertension.

And yet, each of these foods is essential to optimal health, and each is necessary for specific biochemical processes that keep the human body running smoothly. Fats, sugar, and salt are not harmful in themselves. It's the quantity and the forms in which we eat them that can damage our health. That is why fats and sugar are at the top of the Food Guide Pyramid, meaning that they should be consumed in limited quantities. Currently, salt is not at the top of the Food Guide Pyramid. Based on some of the newest research, I believe it will be added soon.

Food manufacturers have seized on the association of fats, sugar, and salt with poor health, and, by modifying foods and playing on our fears, they have completely transformed much of what we eat. Unfortunately, most food manufacturers have not just made our food worse instead of better, they have contributed to the deepening confusion felt by the American public regarding what is healthy and what is not. I'm talking about aggressive marketing of margarine as a substitute for butter or vegetable oils; ceaseless advertising in every medium for fat-free cookies, snack bars, and other snack foods that are densely packed with simple sugars and refined carbohydrates; and promotion of low-salt (and flavorless) foods to people who fear having heart attacks. These alterations in our food and the proliferation of so many unwholesome products have not, for the most part, contributed to a healthier society. Instead, I believe, they have shifted our attention away from whole foods and nutritious meals.

Fat is one of the most complex of all the foods that we eat, at least in terms of the many forms it takes and because there are unanswered ques-

The elements of flavor

Fat, sugar, and salt all contribute to the pleasure of eating and to satiety—the sense of satisfaction you have after you've eaten. Collectively, flavor is a combination of three sensations: taste, smell, and touch. Touch includes the temperature and texture of food in the mouth.

Each of us has more than 10,000 taste buds, most of them on the tongue, with others on the lining of the mouth, tonsils, and back of the throat. Our taste buds are what help us enjoy the four major taste sensations:

- *Sweet,* sensed on the tip of the tongue
- *Sour,* experienced on the sides of the tongue
- *Bitter,* experienced on the back of the tongue
- *Salty,* sensed on the front of the tongue

It's an interesting fact that newborn children have an innate preference for sweetness.

tions about the health benefits of a number of those forms. By contrast, sugar and salt seem relatively straightforward in both their benefits and their drawbacks.

What is the truth about fat, sugar, and salt? And how can we balance good flavor and enjoyment of food with good health? These questions are the focus of this chapter.

FAT: ESSENTIAL TO THE BODY

F*at* is the familiar term we use for lipids, an essential nutrient that the body uses in a number of important ways. In cooking, fats conduct heat, act as a lubricant, add moisture, carry flavors, and help with emulsification by promoting smooth, creamy textures in many food combinations. And they taste good.

What's in dietary lipids?

Lipids are compounds in food and in the body that do not dissolve in water. They are classified into three major types—phospholipids, sterols, and triglycerides. Each has its own chemical makeup and function in the body. In the foods we eat, 95 percent of the lipids are triglycerides, with phospholipids and sterols making up the remaining 5 percent.

Phospholipids
Lecithins are the most common type of phospholipids. In the body, they are important components of the body's cell membranes. Because they have the unique ability to dissolve in both fat and water, phospholipids assist in moving other lipids and fat-soluble hormones and vitamins in and out of cells.

Phospholipids are emulsifiers; that is, they assist in combining fat- and water-soluble substances into a watery solution. The lecithin in foods is used by the food industry as an emulsifier in a wide range of products, such as sauces, mayonnaise, and other salad dressings. Food sources for phospholipids are egg yolks, peanuts, soybeans, liver, and wheat germ.

Sterols

Sterols are a constituent of cell membranes, and they also include bile acids, vitamin D, and adrenal and sex hormones—all crucial to optimal body functioning. The best-known sterol is cholesterol, which your body can make and which is also part of the foods you eat. The cholesterol you get from food derives only from animal sources: dairy products, eggs, meat, fish, and poultry.

Triglycerides

Triglycerides are what we usually mean when we use the word *fat.* They are the major form of fat in the diet and the primary storage form of fat in the body. Their most important functions are to provide enough energy to meet the body's needs every day and, when stored in adipose tissue, to act as an energy reserve. Triglycerides also:

- Help the body use carbohydrates and protein efficiently.
- Protect organs within the body against trauma.
- Provide insulation for body heat.
- Make foods more palatable.
- Assist in the absorption in the GI tract and transport in the blood of fat-soluble vitamins: A, D, E, and K.
- Help satisfy hunger, first by making you feel full when you've finished eating, and second by keeping you full longer because fats are slower to digest than protein and carbohydrates. That's why eating small amounts of fat during a meal can help prevent you from eating too much too often.

Essential fatty acids

Fatty acids are the building blocks of triglycerides and phospholipids. There are numerous fatty acids, and all but two of them are manufactured in sufficient quantity by the body to meet its needs. The two essential fatty acids, which must be supplied in the food we eat at about 3 percent of calories, are *linoleic acid,* an omega-6 fatty acid, and the very similarly named *linolenic acid,* an omega-3 fatty acid. Among other functions, both are necessary for maintaining cell membrane structure and for manufacturing substances that regulate blood pressure, blood clotting, blood lipids, and immune response.

Fatty acids in our food

Oils and fats are nearly always mixtures of the saturated and mono- and polyunsaturated fatty acids described below, but one type usually predominates.

- *Saturated fatty acids,* which come from butter, coconut oil, meat, and poultry, are firm at room temperature. More than 50 percent of these fats is saturated, with the remainder coming from mono- and polyunsaturated fats.
- *Monounsaturated fatty acids* are found in canola, nut, and olive oils. More than 50 percent of them is monounsaturated. They are liquid at room temperature. However, butter, which is solid at room temperature, also contains 30 percent mono- and polyunsaturated fats.
- *Polyunsaturated fatty acids,* which are found in corn, safflower, soybean, and sunflower oils and in most seafood, are soft at room temperature. Over 50 percent of these fats is polyunsaturated.
    Omega-3 fatty acids are highly polyunsaturated and are found in seafood, especially high-fat cold-water fish.
    Omega-6 fatty acids are polyunsaturated. Their food sources are seeds, nuts, grains, meats, and the oils listed under polyunsaturated fatty acids.
- **Trans-***fatty acids* are formed when hydrogen is added to vegetable fats, a process (called hydrogenation) that changes their chemical structure, makes them solid at room temperature, and extends shelf life.

How to identify saturated fats at a glance

Generally speaking, the firmer the fat, the more saturated it is. For example, lard is more saturated than butter; butter is more saturated than safflower oil.

Polyunsaturated fats spoil the most easily and the fastest, so buy only quantities that you know you'll be able to use before they become rancid.

What happens to fats in the body

After a meal, almost all the fat you eat is absorbed in the small intestines and transported through the lymph system. Dietary fat is stored in the body's fat cells, or *adipose tissue*. Adipose cells are unique in their ability to expand and accommodate a virtually unlimited amount of fat. Most of us have enough fat stored already to use as an energy supply for several months, if we take in just a little bit of water.

Fat contains more than twice the energy (calories) of protein and carbohydrates: It provides 9 calories per gram, in contrast to carbohydrates and protein, which contain only 4 calories per gram. This means that fats are an extremely efficient and concentrated storage form of energy, which the body can draw upon as necessary. In fact, throughout the day, most of the energy that you burn comes directly from fat, with smaller amounts of energy from carbohydrates and proteins being used as well.

Fats and carbohydrates interact in crucial ways in the body. Fat can be broken down completely as an energy source only if it is accompanied by the simultaneous use of carbohydrates for energy. When the body lacks sufficient carbohydrates, as would be the case for a person on a high-protein diet, the lipids will fragment into ketone bodies and produce ketosis (see page 110). Fats are also a poor source of glucose, which is essential for brain and nervous system function and for red blood cells.

HOW DIETARY FAT AFFECTS WEIGHT

Obesity has reached epidemic proportions in America and is on the increase worldwide. In the United States, one in two adults and one in four children are overweight. The consequences of obesity, physically and psychologically, are profound. Its causes are complex and not fully understood. Its treatment at present is very difficult, and that is why it is critical to prevent obesity before it begins.

What are the reasons so many Americans are so heavy?

Some of the reasons why

We know that *genetics* plays a major role in the regulation of body weight and energy metabolism, and this promising field is currently under intensive study because the problem of obesity is so immediate. But having the genetic code for a disease or condition does not necessarily mean that you inevitably will get it. Furthermore, gene transformation in nature takes decades if not centuries to happen, and the exponential increase in the obesity has occurred much faster than any evolutionary change in genes could. That is why we know that there are other factors contributing to obesity.

We know that in America *societal factors* are the predominant reason for the great rise in obesity.

The first of these is our increasingly *sedentary lifestyle* in which we spend fewer calories than we take in. Many nutrition professionals believe that lack of exercise is the primary culprit in obesity. In fact, Dr. Jean Mayer, the famous nutritionist for whom our Tufts research center was named, said in 1959, "I am convinced that inactivity is the most important factor explaining the frequency of 'creeping' overweight in modern Western societies." Many nutritionists at the time thought he was crazy and that we were just overeating. Research over the last forty years has shown that he was right!

Obviously, *dietary factors* are also important contributors to obesity; after all, we are what we eat. Most studies—but not all—have shown a positive relationship between dietary fat intake and obesity. In study after study, when people have been put on lower-fat diets, they lose weight. When you eat less fat, you usually eat fewer calories.

Until a couple of years ago, much of the blame for the rise in obesity was attributed to the high percentage of daily calories we get from *dietary fat.* But new evidence suggests that increased fat intake is just part of a larger and more complicated picture.

A decade ago, our dietary fat intake was high. What's intriguing is that, over the last ten years, our fat intake has actually *fallen* to close to suggested levels, but obesity has still continued to soar.

Another major factor is *calorically dense food,* which can be defined as a large amount of calories squeezed into a small volume. Snack bars, muffins, and bagels are examples of calorically dense foods. Many of these commercial food products are low in fat, or even fat-free. But they are packed with carbohydrates, especially simple sugars, and they are very low in water and fiber content. Calorically dense foods contribute to an American diet that overall has a very high glycemic index (see Chapter 4), as research studies are showing us. I believe that these foods are as responsible for obesity as high fat intake and fast foods, or any other factor.

Finally, we know that Americans are eating in *restaurants* more often than ever before, and not just fast-food restaurants. People who eat in restaurants tend to eat fewer fruits and vegetables, and their diets are higher in calories, fat, and saturated fat and lower in fiber than those who eat more often at home. In addition, portion sizes in restaurants (and at home) are exceedingly large, which contributes to the high calorie intake. A recent Tufts University study showed a close correlation between the amount of food eaten at restaurants and body fat.

It will be years before we know the whole story on obesity, but at the very least we can get a start on reversing some of the environmental factors. It may require a long-term national campaign to raise public awareness to the dangers of obesity—a campaign similar to the one waged by the federal government against smoking. Even with public awareness, it will require a conscious effort on the part of every person interested in maintaining a healthy, stable weight to take responsibility for doing so.

HOW DIETARY FAT AFFECTS HEART DISEASE

There are many people who are fat-phobic, but it is important for everyone to understand that dietary fat can have both negative *and* positive effects on your risk for heart disease.

When fats harm the heart

There has been and will continue to be controversy in a number of different fields of nutrition research, but one area has consistently shown detrimental effects on health, and that is the relationship between dietary *saturated fat* and heart disease. The principal reason is that, in many people, saturated fat

Recommended blood cholesterol and triglyceride levels

These are the desirable blood levels of cholesterol and lipids:

Total cholesterol	<200 mg/dL
LDL cholesterol	<130 mg/dL
HDL cholesterol	>35 mg/dL
Triglycerides	<200 mg/dL

What can harm your cholesterol profile
- Genetic predisposition
- High intake of saturated fat, which raises serum cholesterol more than dietary cholesterol does
- Sedentary lifestyle
- Smoking
- Obesity
- Low-fiber diet

How to improve your cholesterol profile
- Replace saturated fats with mono- and polyunsaturated fats.
- Eat foods that contain antioxidants, such as vegetables and fruits.
- Add high-fiber foods to your diet.
- Use alcohol with moderation.
- Lose weight if you are obese.
- Exercise regularly.
- Consult your physician about using appropriate medication.
- The consensus of health and nutrition professionals is that your cholesterol intake should be less than 300 mg/day, whatever your total calorie count is.

intake increases blood cholesterol. *Blood cholesterol* is a major risk factor for heart disease.

There are two primary types of blood cholesterol:

- High-density lipoprotein (HDL, a.k.a. the good cholesterol), which carries cholesterol away from body tissue so it can be excreted. High amounts of HDL are associated with reduced risk of heart disease. A diet that is rich in fruits and vegetables and low in saturated fat, along with moderate alcohol consumption and, especially, exercise, helps to elevate HDL cholesterol.
- Low-density lipoprotein (LDL, a.k.a. the bad cholesterol) circulates through the body. LDL may clog arteries and other blood vessels by forming plaque deposits. High amounts of LDL are associated with the risk of heart disease.

LDL cholesterol in the blood is regulated by diet, heredity, and lifestyle, among other factors. In diet, the amount of saturated fat a person eats is one of the strongest predictors of LDL cholesterol, which has been linked repeatedly with heart disease and premature death in men and women.

Trans-*fatty acids* in particular are the subject of ongoing research—and of controversy—because they are used in so many commercial food products from margarine to baked goods. Although the final word is not yet in, there are numerous studies showing an association between saturated and *trans*-fatty acid intake and heart disease.

In the late 1980s, researchers began to see a correlation between a diet high in *trans*-fatty acids and an elevated LDL-to-HDL ratio in serum cholesterol. Later, in the 1990s, several publications reported that intake of *trans*-fatty acids was associated with an increased risk of heart disease. And more recently, the 1997 Nurses' Health Study (page 49) published in the *New England Journal of Medicine* showed that both saturated and *trans*-fatty acids increased risk of coronary heart disease.

When fats help the heart

The news is not all bad about fat and heart disease. There *is* strong evidence that certain fats reduce your risk of heart disease, and it's backed up by solid scientific research.

Trans-fatty acids: saint or Satan?

The hydrogenation of fats began in the early 1900s. By the 1960s their use had become so widespread that products made with partially hydrogenated fats—margarine, vegetable shortenings, and baked goods, among others—were being consumed, in quantity, in virtually every American household.

Originally, the benefits of partially hydrogenated fats were all to the food industry: decreased costs and longer shelf life. Then, in the true American entrepreneurial spirit (what's good for industry is good for the public), products incorporating hydrogenated fat soon were being touted as healthful, their presumed value being that they reduced the use of saturated fats, such as butter and lard.

But there are health drawbacks to hydrogenation. First, the process tends to make polyunsaturated fats more saturated, diminishing any potential health benefits they may have. And second, the molecules that do remain unsaturated during hydrogenation turn into *trans*-fatty acids. Research has shown that, like saturated fat, *trans*-fatty acids can have adverse health effects on serum cholesterol levels, and that they are also associated with a risk for heart attack.

Are *trans*-fatty acids as detrimental to health as saturated fat? The jury is still out. My recommendation: Keep these fats to a minimum in your diet. Use butter instead of margarine. Your combined intake of saturated and hydrogenated fat should be, at most, one-third of your daily fat consumption, or 10 percent of the total calories you eat.

Currently, manufacturers are not required to list how much *trans*-fatty acids a food contains, but the FDA is trying to change that. In the meantime, be on the lookout for foods with *partially hydrogenated oil* on the ingredients list, and stay away from them if possible.

High trans-*fatty acid foods*
Margarine, cookies, cakes, some dairy and meat products, potato chips, doughnuts, peanut butter, fried foods, and more.

Betty Bought a Bit of Butter . . .

If you've sworn off butter and grudgingly use margarine in its place, you'll be glad to hear that today's choice should be a matter of taste.

Butter made from the milk of cows, goats, yaks, or other animals has a long, interesting, almost regal history, which dates back as far as 2000 B.C. It has been the fat of choice in many cultures for cooking and baking and as a spread and a flavoring. Butter has also been an ingredient in medicines and cosmetics, and put to use in religious worship. By the twelfth century, butter was commonly exported from the Scandinavian countries. In America, the first commercial creamery was built in the United States in 1871 in Iowa.

Several years ago, because of its saturated fat content, butter became the target of a colossal media attack. Butter was the villain menacing your healthy heart, and of course it contributed to obesity, which in turn contributed to type 2 diabetes. Margarine was recommended as the healthy alternative. As a result, a great many people switched to margarine and actually came to fear using butter.

But now, research has shown that the *trans*-fatty acids contained in margarine (and numerous other products) might be just as harmful as the saturated fat found in butter.

Besides confused, where does this leave consumers? Recent research from a laboratory here at Tufts demonstrated that consumption of either butter or classic stick margarine results in the least favorable blood cholesterol (in people with high cholesterol levels) over softer margarines or other oils. The most likely reason for this is that the high levels of saturated fat in butter and the high levels of *trans*-fatty acids in classic stick margarines have equally negative effects on blood cholesterol.

So if you like butter, stick with it. Margarine is no better for you. For butter eaters, there is more positive news. Scientists have discovered that in addition to saturated fat, butter actually contains a health-promoting type of fat—conjugated linoleic acid (CLA), certain types of which have been shown to work as anticancer agents. CLA comprises one third of the fat that is contained in butter.

Does this mean you should generously slather butter on every possible food? Certainly not. Whenever possible, I recommend that you choose olive oil for cooking and sautéing, and use canola oil for baking. But when only butter will do the job—as a spread for pancakes, French toast, and freshly baked bread, and as an ingredient in certain cakes and cookies—use it, and love it. In moderation, butter can be part of the pleasure of eating. We use it in moderation in a number of the recipes contained in this book.

Omega-3 fatty acids

Numerous studies have shown the health-promoting effects of the omega-3 fatty acids that are abundant in cold-water fish such as salmon, sardines, lake trout, albacore tuna, and mackerel, as well as in soybean and canola oils.

A paper published in the *Journal of the American Medical Association* (*JAMA*) in 1995 found that people who did not eat fish at all were at increased risk for sudden cardiac death compared to people who ate fish regularly. Omega-3 fatty acids may reduce the risk of blocked blood vessels and heart attacks by preventing platelets from clotting and sticking to artery walls. These fatty acids may also help prevent hardening of the arteries.

The United States Physician's Health Study, published in *JAMA* in 1998, found that eating fish at least once a week resulted in a 52 percent reduction in the risk of sudden death from heart attacks or stroke. The largest study to date, a randomized, controlled trial of 11,324 subjects who had suffered from a previous stroke, was conducted in Italy and published in *Lancet* in 1999. The subjects were divided into three groups: the first ate a high omega-3 diet (850 mg/day); the second ate the same high omega-3 diet plus a vitamin E supplement; the third group took only a vitamin E supplement. After three and a half years, the data showed that subjects in the first and second groups (high omega-3 diet) had a 20 percent reduction in total mortality and a 45 percent reduction in sudden cardiac death over the third group.

The avocado: a formerly forbidden food

Most of us know avocado as the main ingredient in guacamole. Most of us also know that this luscious fruit contains a considerable amount of fat—nearly 30 grams of fat, or about 300 calories. Not for me, you say.

But wait! Research shows a number of good reasons that avocado has a place in your healthy diet.

- Two-thirds of the fat in an avocado, or 20 grams, is health-promoting monounsaturated fat, the same kind found in olive oil, the kind that has been strongly linked to reduced risk of heart disease.
- Avocados contain beta-sitosterol, a phytoestrogen that animal studies have shown to retard tumor growth and that may lower cholesterol levels by inhibiting absorption of cholesterol from the intestine. Even better, avocados contain four times more beta-sitosterol than other fruits.
- Gluthathione, an antioxidant found in avocados, may help prevent certain types of cancer and heart disease.
- Avocados are a good source of folic acid, which is particularly important for the prevention of neural tube defects and spina bifida. Folic acid has also been found to lower homocysteine levels in the blood, an effect associated with lowered risk of stroke and heart disease (see Chapter 5).
- Avocados are an excellent source of potassium.

I don't suggest that you eat an avocado a day, but like so many formerly forbidden foods, it has a place in your healthy, pleasurable diet. Avocados are now recommended by the Food Guide Pyramid as a source of "good" fat. So next time you're face to face with a guacamole-filled burrito or a sliced avocado and sprouts sandwich on whole-grain bread, go for it!

These results indicate that a diet high in omega-3 fatty acids offers protection against cardiac disease, and that vitamin E had little effect in this high-risk group.

HOW MUCH FAT DO YOU NEED?
WHAT KIND OF FAT SHOULD YOU EAT?

The current recommendation is that no more than 30 percent of your daily calories should come from fat. Americans now get on average 34 percent of their calories from fat. Four percent may seem to be a small difference between the ideal and the real, but over time it adds up to excess calories and excess saturated fat.

Unless you have access to a nutrition evaluation program or keep meticulous track of all the foods you eat and count every last gram of fat, it is very difficult to determine what percent of calories in your diet is coming from fat. Your goal is to get equal amounts, or 10 percent of your calories a day, from saturated, monounsaturated, and polyunsaturated fats. That goal is further complicated because many of the fats you eat are mixtures of these three fats.

Although you cannot arrive at a precise figure for the amount of fat you eat, following the recommendations in the Food Guide Pyramid, you can eat a diet that is likely to be 30 percent fat in the correct proportions. Such a diet is low in processed foods and rich in whole grains and fruits and vegetables. It can include moderate amounts of lean meats, fish, poultry, low-fat or skim dairy products, some butter, with occasional desserts and snacks, such as ice cream, cookies, and other treats. Prudent use of olive oil or other oils rich in monounsaturated fat for cooking and dressings will provide the mono- and polyunsaturated fats you need, and eating cold-water fish a couple of times a week will give you the health-promoting omega-3 fatty acids, which are also polyunsaturated.

Labeling fats and cholesterol

With the plethora of fat jargon on food labels, I thought it would be helpful to have a glossary of fat terms. When choosing reduced-fat products, be wary, because very often sugar and other unhealthful ingredients have been added instead. I encourage you to compare the labels of reduced- and non-fat products with labels on basic, unmodified foods.

This is what the labels mean:

Fat free (also *nonfat, not fat, zero fat*): <0.5 g of fat per serving and no added fats or oil

Low fat: ≤3 g of fat per serving

Less fat: ≤25 percent less fat than comparison foods

Saturated fat free: 1 g or less of saturated fat per serving

Less saturated fat: ≤25 percent less saturated fat than comparison foods

Extra lean: <5 g of fat, 2 g of saturated fat, and 95 mg of cholesterol per serving; and per 100 g of meat, poultry, or seafood

Lean: <10 g of fat, 4.5 g of saturated fat, and 95 mg of cholesterol per serving; and per 100 g of meat

Light: 50 percent or less of the fat in comparison foods

Cholesterol free: less than 2 mg cholesterol and less than 2 mg saturated fat per serving

Low cholesterol: 20 mg or less of cholesterol and less than 2 mg saturated fat per serving

Reduced or less cholesterol: at least 25 percent less cholesterol than comparison foods, and less than 2 mg saturated fat

Fat replacements

Food producers use a variety of fat-replacement agents in food. Although they decrease the fat content, not all of them are calorie free because many of them have their own calorie content and because extra sugar often is added to make the foods more palatable. The replacements are used in such foods as cheese, cookies, salad dressings and mayonnaise, ice cream, sour cream, candy, and potato chips.

Some of the fat replacements include those that are protein-based (Simplesse), carbohydrate-based (modified starch, dextrin, cellulose, gums), and fat-based (Olestra, Salatrim).

Once fat replacements are used in a food, the food is changed, not just in its fat content but in many other ways as well. I recommend that you stay away from these highly processed substances and stick with whole foods. The long-term health effects of these substitutes are not known. As we have seen with *trans*-fatty acids, it takes decades of research to fully understand how they affect our health.

I remember once at a nutrition industry dinner being served a "cheesecake" that was fat- and sugar-free—it tasted awful. In fact, I had only one bite because I couldn't begin to imagine all the chemicals that had been crammed into that altered food!

Fats are so important nutritionally and in cooking that, however controversial they are, they will continue to have a profound effect on the health of all Americans. The challenge is getting the right amount and type of fat for optimal health. Once again, awareness of what is in the food we eat and our pleasure in eating it is the healthy and enjoyable approach to fats.

SUGAR

Part of our genetic heritage is an inborn taste for sweet foods, and our diet has always included them, starting from the very beginning of human life when we foraged for berries and other fruits.

Honey was the primary sweetener in Europe until about 1500, when refined sugar cane came into greater use. Even then, it was still a luxury and used more often in medicines (just a spoonful was needed to make them go down) than as a sweetener for food. But by the eighteenth century, cookbooks appeared that were devoted entirely to the use of sugar in various confections. And by the eighteenth century, millions of Africans were enslaved for the purpose of cultivating sugar cane in the new European colonies in the Caribbean.

The creation of new technology during the industrial revolution made refined sugar cane affordable in most middle-class and wealthy households by the early nineteenth century. Meanwhile, the first full-scale refinery for beet sugar was established outside of Paris by order of Napoleon. Today about 40 percent of the world supply of sugar comes from beets, much of them grown and refined in the United States.

Sources of sugar: natural and added

Whether natural or added, sugar is a carbohydrate that comes in the following forms:

Monosaccharides: glucose, galactose, fructose

Disaccharides: maltose (glucose + glucose), lactose (glucose + galactose), sucrose (glucose + fructose)

These simple sugars are absorbed in the gut and for the most part transformed into glucose within the body and stored in muscle and other organs as glycogen, or used as an energy source. For more information about the metabolism of carbohydrates and the glycemic index, see Chapter 4.

Moderate amounts of both naturally occurring and added sugars are part of any healthy diet. Sugar adds flavor, aroma, color, body, and texture to innumerable foods. Simple sugars are all the same, whether naturally occurring or added. But I believe it is important to eat more of the healthy foods containing naturally occurring sugars. In themselves, those foods are so much more nutritious than many of the foods containing added sugars that it's no contest—we know what to choose.

Naturally occurring sugars are inherent in many of the foods we eat: fruits and vegetables (in which the sugar is produced by photosynthesis), grains, milk, and fermented alcoholic beverages.

Although the sugar in fruit juices occurs naturally and does provide many of the vitamins and minerals found in the fruits themselves, fruit juice in general does not supply the fiber of the whole fruit. Many drinks, such as fruit-based beverages, cocktails, and others, are not pure juice, and they tend to be loaded with added sugars, which you can discover easily by reading the nutrition facts labels.

Added sugars usually originate in a natural source, such as sugar cane or sugar beets or maple trees, but they are manufactured for the express

Sugar myths

Some firmly held beliefs about sugar seem to make sense because we've heard them repeated so often, but in fact they are not true. For instance:

- Brown and turbinado sugars are not healthier than white sugar—they are all equal in nutritional value. Molasses, on the other hand, has a significant amount of calcium and other minerals, which make it healthier.
- Sugar does not cause diabetes, although it can be a contributory factor.
- Eaten in moderation, sugar does not cause obesity, and neither does fat. It is extra-large portion sizes, the great number of foods with added sugars that we eat, and lack of physical activity that are much more important in contributing to obesity.
- Sugar (especially in chocolate) does not cause acne. The condition is thought to occur in teenagers because of the hormonal changes they undergo.
- "This food has no sugar. It doesn't taste sweet at all." In fact, beer, wine, and liquor all have high sugar contents. One cup of grape or apple juice contains more simple sugar (albeit naturally occurring sugar) than ¾ cup of frosted flakes or ice cream.

purpose of adding sweetness to food. The dry forms of added sugar are: brown sugar, granulated sugar, cane sugar (or table or white sugar), raw sugar, turbinado sugar, confectioner's sugar, and maple sugar. Syrups are: honey, corn syrup, corn sweeteners, maple syrup, high-fructose corn syrup (used in manufacturing processed foods and beverages), dextrose, and molasses.

Life is sweet: Is there a place for candy in a healthy diet?

Halloween is one of my children's favorite annual rituals. It ranks right up there with Christmas. I love the festive event too, but I must say that I do not enjoy having a glut of candy around the house for days to come. However, I do believe that candy and sweets have a place in most people's diets—the trick (and the treat) is to find the right balance. There is no doubt that if you are on a weight-control or weight-loss diet, you need to keep high-calorie snacks and candy to a minimum. But if you are weight stable, candy can be enjoyed in moderation. The good news is that research is showing us that candy can be health-promoting.

- One recent study of Harvard alumni demonstrated that the group of men in the study who totally abstained from eating candy also had the highest mortality rate. The lowest mortality was in men who consumed candy from one to three times per month to one to two times per week. (Those who ate candy three or more times a week had higher mortality.) Men who ate some candy lived almost a year longer than those who ate no candy at all.
- Chocolate, particularly good-quality dark chocolate (a high-sugar food) contains the flavonoid catechin, an antioxidant. Catechin is a phytochemical—also found in tea—that is thought to have a role in reducing the risk for heart disease and cancer.
- Another study of chocolate, published in *Lancet* in 1996, showed that cacao powder extract is a powerful antioxidant for reducing the oxidation of LDL cholesterol.

The bottom line is that moderate candy consumption—especially of chocolate—seems to promote health and reduce mortality. I also strongly believe that a little treat every now and then sure tastes good.

The drawbacks of eating too many sweets

You are likely to be familiar with the drawbacks of eating too many sweets, but it is worth reviewing.

- Sugars contribute to tooth decay. That includes sugars added to foods as well as from processed grains such as white flour or pasta. The stickier the carbohydrate the more likely that it will contribute to tooth decay. Bacteria in your mouth and around your teeth thrive on carbohydrates, and after feeding on them, these bacteria produce acids that cause decay. Brushing after every meal and snack and flossing daily will help prevent these acids from forming.
- By itself, sugar does not cause diabetes. However, the combination of high sugar intake with low dietary fiber does put a person at elevated risk for the development of type 2 diabetes.

Does sugar cause hyperactivity in children?

As a mother and a nutrition scientist, I have followed the sugar-hyperactivity debate for years. Most parents believe that there is a link between sugar consumption and hyperactivity in their children. There has been intensive, carefully controlled research over the past two decades on this issue, and almost all of the research has shown that no such link exists.

I believe this research, but as a mother I also know that my children do much better behaviorally and academically when they have a well-rounded diet that has a minimum of high-sugar snacks. Think about how you feel when you have eaten poorly for several days at a time—you feel awful, and you're unproductive. I think children are affected the same way.

Sugar may not cause hyperactivity, but too much sugar eaten too often can make you feel lousy, and I am sure it makes your children feel lousy too.

- In general, high sugar intake in and of itself is not a risk factor for heart disease. But studies in 1995 and 1998, both published in the *American Journal of Clinical Nutrition,* found that high sugar consumption does increase blood lipids and puts a person at increased risk for heart disease. High intake of refined sugar together with a lack of fiber in the diet can put a person at elevated risk for both diabetes and heart disease.

What the sugar labels mean

To date, the FDA does not require food manufacturers to distinguish between naturally occurring sugars and the sugars they add during processing.

Sugar-free: <0.5 g of sugar

Calorie-free: less than 5 calories

Reduced or *less sugar:* at least 25 percent less than found in comparison foods

No added sugar; without added sugar; no sugar: no sugars added during processing and and packing

Low sugar: may NOT be used on food labels

High-sugar foods

Cookies, cakes, pies, candy, soda pop, jelly, fruit drinks, syrups, honey, beer, wine, hard liquor.

Artificial sweeteners

In my opinion, unless you are diabetic there is no place in the diet for artificial sweeteners. Many people use a packet of artificial sweetener in their morning hot beverage. A teaspoon of sugar has only 15 calories, which is negligible. There is nothing wrong with using a little sugar or honey in your tea or coffee! Artificial sweeteners have also found their way into ice cream, yogurts, dressings, and countless other "sugar-free" products. I encourage you to stay away from these foods. Stick with the natural variety. If you eat wholesomely throughout the day, you will not eat too much sugar!

The FDA has approved three sweeteners as safe:

- *Aspartame:* Brand names Nutrasweet and Equal; it is 180 to 200 times sweeter than sugar. Aspartame is a compound of two amino acids, aspartic acid and phenylalanine, which occur naturally in fruits, vegetables, meat, and milk. People with phenylketonuria (PKU) should not use it, and foods containing aspartame must be labeled. It loses its sweetness when used in baking and cooking. Although some people claim to be allergic to aspartame, no dangerous symptoms have been noted. One of the most studied of all food additives, it has been approved for use in over a hundred nations.
- *Saccharin:* Brand name Sweet 'N Low, it is three hundred times sweeter than sugar and is made from a substance that occurs naturally in grapes. Saccharin has been marketed since the nineteenth century. However, in the late 1970s the FDA proposed banning saccharin because of research showing that exceedingly high doses increased the risk of bladder cancer in rats. The FDA withdrew that proposal in 1991, although products containing saccharin must carry a warning label, "Use of this product may be hazardous to your health. This product contains saccharin, which has been determined to cause cancer in laboratory animals." Despite this label, saccharin is considered safe when used at moderate levels. It retains its sweetness during cooking and baking and has been approved for use in over a hundred countries.
- *Acesulfame-K:* Brand name Sunette, acesulfame-K was discovered in the late 1960s and approved by the FDA in 1988. It is two hundred times sweeter than sugar and, because of its aftertaste, it is often combined with other sweeteners. Sunette retains its sweetness during cooking and baking.

SALT

Salt, or sodium chloride, is essential to human life and it has always been prized. In the Old Testament, salt is an offering to God. The Romans called it *sal* after their god of health, and our word *salary* comes from Roman *salarium,* the allowance paid to Roman soldiers to buy salt.

The culinary value of salt cannot be overstated. It is used as a flavoring in itself (we have a specialized taste sensation for it), to heighten other flavors or sweeten bitter tastes, and as a preservative. Even when we cannot identify the taste of salt in a particular food, we immediately know when it is absent—have you ever tasted bread or soup made without salt?

Salt in the body

Salt is a compound of two essential elements, sodium and chloride. Your body cannot function without salt. Among its functions:

- Salt assists in nerve transmission and muscle contractions.
- It is vital to maintaining electrolyte balance by controlling the passage of fluids in and out of the cells; it helps move nutrients into cells and transports waste away from them.
- Salt assists with regulating blood pressure.

Salt in your food—how much do you need, how much do you get?

The aggregate of foods that you eat usually provides more sodium than your body needs. The recommended daily amount of sodium for a normally active person is 2,400 mg or less. As a visual aid, think of a teaspoon of table salt: It contains 2,300 mg of sodium. Most Americans consume 4,000 to 6,000 mg a day. This discrepancy of 1,600 to 3,600 mg a day is not due to the intake of salt that occurs naturally in unseasoned food, nor is it because of salt added during cooking or at the table—it is salt added by the food industry to processed foods.

Only athletes and other people who are very active physically need more than 2,400 mg a day. Because athletes need to eat more than sedentary people, they almost always get enough salt. However, a person who exercises strenuously in excessively hot conditions will need to replenish electrolytes and salts during and after exercise.

How salt intake can affect your health

High sodium intake may precipitate high blood pressure in genetically predisposed salt-sensitive people. Such individuals are most likely to be African American, diabetic, hypertensive, over 50 years old, or people with chronic renal disease. According to the American Dietetic Association, 30 percent of Americans have sodium-sensitive blood pressure. This means that two-thirds of the population are not salt-sensitive and do not have to drastically restrict their salt intake. At present there is no easy test for salt sensitivity that can predict who will develop hypertension.

Some people, especially nutritionally conscious older adults, are excessively worried about salt and hypertension. As a result, they limit their salt intake to such an extent that they take in too little salt and experience hypotension, or low blood pressure. There is no need—in fact, it is unhealthy—to exclude salt entirely from your diet. The key is moderation.

What salt/sodium labels mean

As with sugar, these values are for all the sodium contained in a particular food, with no distinction drawn between naturally occurring salt and salt added by the food processor.

Sodium or *salt free:* <5 mg of sodium per serving
Very low sodium: 35 mg or less per serving
Low sodium: 140 mg or less per serving
Reduced or *less sodium:* at least 25 percent less than comparison foods
Light: low-calorie, low-fat food with a 50 percent reduction in sodium
Light in sodium: no more that 50 percent of the sodium of comparison
   foods

High-sodium foods

Processed foods, especially canned soups, beans, vegetables, and other canned foods; soy sauce or tamari; table salt; pickled foods; olives; sauerkraut; processed meats such as sausages, bologna, salamis, and hot dogs;

ham; corned beef; anchovies; caviar; canned tuna; herring; sardines; smoked salmon; regular canned bouillon; Worcestershire and barbecue sauces; catsup and mustard and other condiments.

This list only touches the surface. To learn the sodium content of many more foods, check out the FDA sodium website listed in Resources. If you look at the food label on a product, it might surprise you to discover that foods that taste salty don't necessarily contain a lot of sodium. Rice Krispies and cornflakes have over twice the amount of sodium as a comparable amount (by weight) of potato chips or salted peanuts. The two latter foods wear their salt on their sleeves—it's all on the surface. In the breakfast cereals, sodium is blended into the product with numerous other additives, flavor enhancers, etc.

Strategies for cutting your sodium intake

- Season your foods with very moderate amounts of salty condiments, or none, and use salt-free spices, fruits such as lemon, lime, and orange, and fresh or dried herbs.
- Use moderate amounts of salt in cooking, or use none at all whenever possible.
- Try low-salt and salt-free products, such as salt-free bouillon. Salt substitutes, on the other hand, taste really awful.
- Choose fresh over processed foods whenever possible.

The good, the bad, and the ugly—that sums up fats, sugars, and salt. They are necessary to a healthy body and to a pleasurable diet. In fact, several fats are critical to optimal health—oils from fish, for example. But, as we all know, when eaten in excess, fats, sugars, and salts can be harmful factors that contribute to heart disease, obesity, diabetes, and tooth decay. A diet rich in whole grains, fruits, and vegetables and moderate in fats, sugar, and salt is the right mix. If you eat only a limited amount of processed foods and have a varied diet, you will be assured of getting all the good nutrition you need.

CHAPTER 10

What's for Dinner?

Keep the Good Stuff on Hand

❖

How many times have you come home from work, hungry and tired, and found no food in the house to use for a decent dinner—so you settle for cold cereal and milk?

I haven't had cereal for dinner in a long time, but I do find, most weeks, that by Wednesday or Thursday our supply of fresh foods is quite low. Most often what we do is find ways to use some of the longer-lasting fresh vegetables in combination with our store of canned, dried, and frozen foods to make something wholesome and tasty for dinner.

I know there are people who like to shop every day for fresh foods, for bread, for the best buys, for that very special kind of spice or cheese or chocolate—it's part of the way they think about food and cooking. But for many of you, even if you wanted to spend the time, you don't have it to spend. In my family we do our major food shopping and a lot of the cooking on the weekend. Midweek, we make quick trips to the markets, when we have time, to fill in the blanks. It's taken a while, but we've (almost) learned to think ahead, and by now we usually have enough on hand to make nutritious meals throughout the week.

Of course, like many American families, we also plan to have leftovers. It takes time to cook the stews and casseroles that my family loves, so we usually cook enough to last for two or more meals. We often cook more grains, beans, even fresh vegetables than we can eat at one meal, because we know we will use them the next day in new combinations, with new seasonings, and with fresh additions. If you look at the recipes for Curried Brown Rice Salad (page 218), Oma's Easter Grain Pie (page 236), or Fish and Corn Chowder (page 199), you'll get an idea of the way we use leftovers.

What's for dinner, Mom?

Each person's needs, food preferences, budget, and kitchen space are individual. These are the food staples in *my* pantry.

Dairy   It needs to be fresh—that's what to look for first. In our community we are fortunate to have a local dairy that delivers milk in the old milk bottles as well as fresh eggs, ice cream, yogurt, and other dairy products. Everything tastes very fresh, and it's also nice to know that these foods come from a place that I actually know and can visit. Dairy products in the stores are marked with the last date of sale, so buy the item with the date furthest in the future. Get just enough to last you until your next scheduled shopping trip. I also try to go to the local cheese shop on the weekends to buy some good imported cheese for snacks throughout the week and Parmesan, which we grate fresh for pasta.

Grains   I keep whole-wheat and unbleached all-purpose flours, several kinds of rice, barley, oatmeal, couscous (for those truly quick meals), grits, and a few other grains on hand. I prefer to use organic grains, but if they're not available, I use what is. I date grains and store them for a month or two at most because they can spoil. I know it sounds crazy, but we have a supply of whole corn kernels because we have cornmeal pancakes several days a week, and my children love to grind the corn for them—and of course the pancakes taste better, too. We have whole-grain breads and crackers as well as several types of pasta in the house—the shapes my children like best.

Fruits Apples, citrus fruits, and some others keep well for a few days, usually in the refrigerator. Several fruits, such as berries, we buy in season, or, in a pinch, frozen to serve over waffles and cereals. My family loves dried fruits—apricots, dates, figs, cranberries, raisins, prunes, currants, and apples—and we always have some in the house for snacks and cooking.

Vegetables I can't imagine looking in my refrigerator and not finding carrots, celery, peppers, and some kind of salad greens; can't imagine looking in my vegetable bin and not seeing onions and garlic. We eat a lot of fresh vegetables, but then we always have something in the freezer: broccoli, peas, corn, spinach, and others.

Dried lentils, which cook in only twenty-five minutes, and other dried beans don't take up much space. But when we don't have the time, canned beans of every variety are useful. And the most indispensable of all canned vegetables—tomatoes—are always in my pantry ready for a quick sauce.

Fish, poultry, and meat We usually eat these three proteins fresh on weekends and early in the week, then eat a mostly vegetarian diet the rest of the week. I think it's a good balance nutritionally, and very practical in terms of shopping. Eggs, canned tuna, and sardines are part of the larder, too.

Chicken and vegetable stocks I don't love it, but for soups, stews, cooking grains, sauces, and so on, canned chicken broth has its uses. Try to find a brand without too chemical a taste. If a brand you like is too salty, dilute it with water. There are now several kinds of low-fat and fat-free chicken broths, both organic and nonorganic, as well as some moderately priced vegetable broths packed in nonrefrigerated, aseptic, sale-dated cartons. Many supermarkets carry them, and they are available in most health food stores. If more than one brand is available, you might want to taste-test them to see which is most pleasing to your palate.

Nuts and seeds Both are healthy, if highly caloric, snacks—good roasted and tossed into salads, used in cookies and cakes, pilafs, and innumerable other recipes, too. I keep a few kinds on hand—I like almonds, and my husband and kids like mixed nuts—and buy the rest when I need them for a specific recipe. We always have sunflower seeds in the house. I pan-roast them and add them to salads and to the Sunday-morning waffle mix. Rancid seeds and nuts look just like the fresh ones, so buy from a reliable source and, if possible, taste before you buy. I put them into airtight containers, date them, and store them in a dark place if I'm keeping them for only a week or two, and in the freezer if there's room for them.

Soy foods   We buy edamame frozen, both shelled and in the pod. It's quite rare at the moment to find them fresh. Tofu lasts for several days, submerged in water and kept in the refrigerator. Our family eats tofu the way many other families eat hamburger—we have it several nights a week. Served with brown rice, beans, and vegetables, it's a delicious midweek meal, and easy to prepare.

Oils   We use olive oil for dressings and cooking, canola and safflower oils for other cooking, and butter for baking, toast, and occasionally for vegetables and eggs. We never use margarine. Sesame, soy, peanut, corn, and hazelnut oils are also useful, but I usually buy them only for specific recipes. Oil becomes rancid if kept too long, if left uncovered, and if not stored in a cool dark place. If oil smells or tastes "off," throw it out.

Vinegar   I'm something of a nut about vinegar for flavoring stews, deglazing pans, and preparing salad dressings, so I keep quite a few around: red wine, balsamic, sherry, raspberry, rice wine, and cider are the ones I cram onto their own little shelf. Most people make do with fewer than these.

Sweet things   We have what you'd expect—honey, molasses, white and brown sugars, a few jams and jellies, marmalade. My husband always has some good chocolate hidden away in the pantry—if the kids or I look hard enough, we can usually find it!

Baking   Baking powder, baking soda, cream of tartar, chocolate chips, baking (unsweetened) chocolate, semisweet or bittersweet chocolate, cocoa, vanilla, almond, and other extracts are my baking basics.

Spices and condiments   We keep salt (coarse kosher salt); black pepper-corns, far too many spices, which I date when I bring them home (but they still always get old before I throw them out); bay leaves; a few dried herbs (fortunately, many more fresh ones are available year round in supermarkets); two kinds of mustard; catsup; mayonnaise; tamari; and mild salsa.

Beverages   We like fresh and frozen juices, tea, frozen coffee beans for guests because neither my husband nor I drink coffee, sparkling water, beer, wine, and cider. Only when my mother comes to visit do we have sodas in the house, and my children can't wait.

Specialty foods   I am a pretty basic cook, so I don't keep many specialty foods on hand. I know others do, and these can include anything from hot sauce to capers, dried porcini mushrooms, olives, anchovies, green pepper-corns, chutney—and many more.

Cooking equipment . . . a few of my favorite things

Years ago, a friend who was a gifted cook told me that all you really needed in order to produce a creditable meal was a bowl, a spoon, a knife, and a pot. How true, I thought, as my kitchen is pretty basic. Later I visited his home and saw how far, wide, and deep the abyss was between his words and his own snazzily equipped palace, where he prepared an exquisite meal. I was humbled once again, but differently.

Some of our tools have special meaning for us. Used over time and used lovingly and well, a tool can become a ritual object, part of a repeated cere-monial act, and it takes on a life of its own. I particularly love some of the cookware that I have picked up at secondhand shops, like the battered stove-top baker, which makes the best baked potatoes without heating up the whole house. I love the shallow wooden chopping bowl and the old carbon steel chopper with a wooden handle that I still use for small quantities of nuts or herbs. I love particularly the well-seasoned cast-iron skillets, which I use every day.

You know far better than I what you need in order to produce a creditable meal in your own kitchen, so I'll tell you just a very few of the things that I can't do without.

- Good knives: paring, carving, large chef's, medium chef's, bread, and tomato. It is so much more efficient and pleasurable to cook with sharp knives.
- Knife sharpener: I use a specialty diamond whetstone that was given to me by the woman who makes them. It keeps the knives sharp as the dickens (see the Resources section).
- Spoons, spatulas, and scrapers: lots of them—wooden, metal, plastic, icing spatulas, rubber scrapers, all sizes.
- Cast-iron skillets: My mother used them, I use them, and I suppose my children will too, to fry, sauté, stew, roast, and broil. Handsome and indestructible.
- Stock pot: good for stock, large batches of soup, steaming corn, and making pasta.
- Vegetable steamer.
- Double boiler.
- Microplane grater for grating citrus zest, nutmeg, and cheese: I think of mine as the greater grater. Get one with a rubber handle. They work miraculously well.
- Food processor, preferably with an auxiliary blade that does fine shredding.
- Blender, still an invaluable tool.
- Parchment paper: for lining cookie sheets and cake pans. Simplifies your life.
- Self-adhesive labels; Sharpies (indelible markers).

That's it. While I don't have any nonstick pans, I know that many people like them. If you do get some, make sure they are good quality. Inevitably, your kitchen preferences will vary from mine. But whatever your cooking style, it helps to have the right tools for the job.

Sharing the honors, sharing the work

Weekends are when my whole family cooks together. I grew up cooking with my mother and other relatives, and, lucky for me, so did my husband. Now, when it's possible, we cook together, and even if only one of us is doing the actual cooking, the other is usually in the kitchen, giving advice (thanks!) and lending a hand.

We've found that meals are always more pleasurable to prepare and eat when we work as a team, and now our children have begun helping out, too. My son loves to grind corn for pancakes, my daughters bake with us and are learning to make special family dishes.

Does this sound like a Norman Rockwell *Saturday Evening Post* cover? Believe me, not every meal we put on the table evokes cries of rapture—very often it's "Spaghetti again?" It's having family meals together that counts for us. Although we can't manage it every night, we try very hard.

That's how it is in my household, but maybe not in yours. There are so many living arrangements possible for each of us—the ones we choose and the ones we find ourselves in—and there are even more ways that people eat their meals. But everyone has to eat, every day.

Maybe you eat alone most of the time—or with eight other people; you may do all the cooking for yourself or your family; you may share the cooking chores with others; or you may simply order up occasionally from a local restaurant or pizzeria. Whatever the circumstances, try to commit yourself to providing tasty, nourishing meals for yourself and anyone else who's eating with you.

Even if you don't like to shop and cook, you still can devise your own strategies—ones that work for your situation—to make sure you have enjoyable, wholesome meals.

BE PREPARED

The week before I wrote this chapter I spent six days in France doing some work for Tufts University. We were at the Tufts campus in Talloires, in the Alps, about an hour outside Geneva. Besides hiking in the

When you're on your own

If you're a single woman who's raising her children alone, whatever their ages, it can be singularly difficult making it all work. Often it's the meals that get lost in the shuffle—you have to figure out how to get food on the table and then how to get everyone to sit down and eat it. Your strategies probably include lots of advance planning—buying at food stores that deliver, depending on cooked food from delis, supermarkets, and the takeout counters of healthy restaurants (not just pizzerias), and eating out occasionally.

When you're raising children, in a one- or a two-parent household, nothing can replace the family meal in terms of quality of life. Research has shown that sitting down around the table together at mealtime, without the television on, is positively associated with better school grades, fewer disciplinary problems, lower obesity rates in children, and a better sense of well-being. Even when kids eat fast and are gone, even a ten-minute dinner can make a difference.

Recently, I was talking to an acquaintance, Sylvia, who is bringing up her daughter alone. Every night they have a sit-down dinner at the table, very often spaghetti because her daughter is not adventurous about eating new foods. Sylvia has an interesting way to enrich dinner. Once or twice a week they have dinner with her daughter's best friend and her best friend's mother, either at Sylvia's apartment or at her friend's apartment or at a restaurant. That way the family circle is enlarged, and the weekly meals are occasions everyone can look forward to.

mountains every afternoon, one of the most memorable parts of the trip was the incredible fresh food.

None of the food we ate came in plastic bags or was more than a day old. The bread was baked fresh every morning. The yogurt came in little ceramic pots. Even the cheese was from cows that we walked past up in the mountains. The hardest transition coming back to the States was reentering the world of American food. Very few of us have the opportunity or time to gather fresh foods each day for a delicious, wholesome meal. But there *are some* strategies that can help even the busiest person get a good meal to the table.

Plan ahead

Okay, you *think ahead,* and what you think is: I don't want to cook tonight. But if you *plan ahead,* you might just be able to do it, and most of the food might be right there in the fridge waiting for you. For example, our family likes brown rice—but brown rice (and other whole grains) takes at least twice as long to cook as white rice. So what I try to do when I first come home in the evening, is put on the brown rice. Then I catch up with the kids or take a short walk with the dogs to unwind, and then I get dinner going. By the time dinner is ready, the rice is cooked. I always cook more than we're going to eat that night, so that I have brown rice for the next day's meal.

I much prefer to use real dried beans instead of canned ones whenever I'm able to—but who has time to cook dried beans? The trick here is to just think about putting up the beans to soak the night before so they'll be ready the next day. The actual time you spend in preparation is no longer than for other foods—you just need to make the plan. Some people I know leave themselves notes, some get their children or partners to either do the prep work or to remind them to do it; others say the words out loud, but very low: "I've got to soak the beans tonight."

Prepare more than you need

It is so luxurious to go to the refrigerator and find a big bag of lettuce that has been washed already and needs only a salad dressing before it goes to the table, or to see a tightly sealed bag of chopped vegetables just waiting to be steamed. Many foods can be prepared well ahead of time, so while you're washing and chopping greens and other vegetables, wash and chop more than you need and store them for tomorrow's meal. Serving the same vegetables two days in a row is fine, especially if you cook them in different ways.

Cook more than you need

Leftovers are a way of life in our family. As I write this, I can hear my children's groans in the next room as they contemplate yet another day of vegetable stew. Leftovers seem to me the ultimate in advance planning, from whole meal leftovers like stews and casseroles, to leftovers that can be recycled into other dishes, most notably grains and vegetables, which are such versatile foods. We use leftover grains for dishes ranging from waffles—we just throw them into the batter—to savory rice puddings to salads to stir-fries to desserts, or we just reheat them in the double boiler. Leftover cooked vegetables go into salads, frittatas, grain dishes, whatever comes to mind and to hand when I open the refrigerator door.

Use your freezer

I am working hard to use my freezer more. I love to visit my mother, who always has a great meal waiting for her in the freezer—a treasure trove of stocks, chicken carcasses, vegetables and fruits, nuts and seeds, cooked foods such as soups and stews, bread, butter, ice cream—it's a long list. After many years of coming across nameless mystery foods at the back of the freezer, I'm starting to learn not just to pack and seal everything carefully but to label and date it as well. I try to take an inventory of frozen foods every few months so I can either use or dispose of older items. Two-year-old chicken (which I unearthed a while ago) is inedible and takes up valuable space.

Splurge on home delivery

When I grew up in the mid-1960s, the local grocer in our small Pennsylvania town would deliver groceries. We didn't use the service in our family, but one of our neighbors did, and I thought it was so cool. Now, supermarkets in many metropolitan areas have delivery service that is coordinated through a website from which you can order your food, and presto! It shows up whenever you need more food. I have a number of colleagues who use such services because when both spouses work, there's almost no time for shopping. For these people, getting home deliveries means they have fresh food available all the time and won't have to resort to fast food. If it's an option for you, try out home delivery, see how fresh the vegetables and fruits are, see if it works for you.

Order out

Most people living in urban areas, and some living in the suburbs, have the luxury of ordering from a local restaurant and getting a tasty, nutritious meal delivered quickly—usually something you wouldn't cook yourself or bring home from the grocery freezer shelves. My family orders out a few times a month from a local Chinese restaurant. The food is fresh and my kids love it. When my husband and I go out for dinner we usually order pizza for the kids—the kids are thrilled and I am, too, because I don't have to eat it (I am not a pizza fan). Our community is small and doesn't have a lot of options. I am sure if I lived in an area with a greater range of takeout, I would take advantage of it.

As in most households, our family doesn't eat splendid meals every day—we get into those familiar ruts just as every other family does—but we keep working at it. And just like every other family, with our busy schedules and after-school activities, simply having the energy to put together a wholesome meal is not always easy, but with a little bit of planning and creativity you can do it!

CHAPTER 11

What's in Food Today?

❖

Our choice of foods has changed dramatically over the last century. In 1900, most of our food was still grown or produced locally, and it was rare that anything from outside the community appeared on our tables except for staples such as wheat flour, sugar, coffee and tea, and luxuries such as imported wines and chocolate.

Since then there has been a remarkable increase in the number of foods available to us on an everyday basis. In very broad terms, there are three reasons for this. The first is improvements in the transportation and preservation of food. The second is a new sophistication in this country about foods from other cultures, much of it due to a century of wars in which American soldiers fought overseas and an influx of people from many countries who were forced to leave their homelands and settle here. The third reason is American wealth: We have more disposable income to spend on food.

As I mentioned in Chapter 1, only fifty years ago there were on average 2,000 different food products in a supermarket. Then, in the 1980s, that number increased to 5,000 or so food products. Now, at the beginning of the new millennium, most supermarkets carry more than 40,000 different food products from which we can choose—superstores carry more than 60,000! No wonder shopping is such a daunting task.

Few of us know where these foods come from or how they are grown or how they have been stored or what has been added to them or if they are healthy for us or whether they will increase the risk for chronic disease.

There are quite a number of terms used to describe the foods that have been cropping up recently. *Organic* and *genetically engineered* are of special significance to anyone who wants to eat a healthy diet and feed a healthy family.

WHAT ABOUT ORGANIC FOOD?

By now you know that I'm a big believer in whole foods. I'm also a believer in organic foods—but I'm not a zealot about them. I buy organic or locally grown food whenever I can, but I buy conventionally grown foods as well. What my family eats depends on what's available, how it looks, feels, and smells.

For the most part, research has shown us that the vitamin and mineral content of organically grown food is no greater than that of conventional food. But there are other reasons that I buy organic. First of all, it is grown without harmful substances such as pesticides and herbicides, which can find their way into our bodies and into the soil in which food is grown.

I believe that organic foods taste better. There is nothing quite as delicious as the fresh vegetables and fruits grown on my brother-in-law's farm in New Hampshire. I have never tasted a better carrot, a sweeter beet, or more tender spinach. If you haven't eaten organic fruits and vegetables, I encourage you to try them, especially when they are in season and freshly harvested.

Organically grown foods are much healthier for our environment because they require agricultural methods that enrich rather than deplete the soil. These methods promote biological diversity and the recycling of resources through crop rotation, rotational grazing, the planting of cover crops, intercropping, composting, recycling, tilling, and adding minerals to crops.

The primary goal of organic agriculture is to optimize the health and productivity of interdependent communities of soil life, plants, animals, and people. This may sound utopian and impractical, but in fact, organic farming happens to be one of the fastest growing sectors of American agriculture. The USDA estimates the retail sales value of organic food in 1999 was approximately $6 billion. The number of organic farmers is increasing by about 12 percent a year and now stands at over 12,000 nationwide, most of them small-scale producers.

What does the label "Certified Organic" mean?

The principal guidelines for organic food production are the use of materials and practices that enhance the ecological balance of natural systems and that integrate the parts of the farming system into an ecological whole.

Federal legislation governing organic agriculture was passed in 1990 with the Organic Foods Production Act, which required the USDA to develop guidelines and regulations for organic food production. By December 1997, the USDA had published a proposed set of rules for labeling and opened up those rules for public comment. As you can imagine, almost 300,000 people and organizations commented on the rules, which have since been revised. By the time this book is published, new federal laws, administered by the National Organic Program (NOP) of the USDA, will be in effect. These laws mandate a single national standard for labeling organic foods. Individual states are still permitted to set their own standards, but they must be at least as rigorous as those set by the federal government.

California has long been a leader in the certification of organically grown and produced foods. By 1990, the California Organic Foods Act was passed, and for over a decade it was the standard referred to by organic food producers on their labels with the words "Certified organically grown and processed in accordance with the California Organic Foods Act of 1990." Many organic products produced before the federal law went into effect may be labeled with this phrase.

New federal organic labeling laws

Some of the broad areas covered by the new labeling standards require the prohibition of genetically engineered foods, sewage sludge, and irradiation in the production of organic foods. Farmers raising organic livestock cannot use antibiotics for growth purposes and are required to give the animals 100 percent organic feed. Livestock cannot be totally confined and must graze in pastureland.

These laws help consumers understand the food they are buying and help the farmers market their foods more effectively. Labeling requirements are based on the percentage of organic ingredients in the product:

- *100% organic*   The food must contain 100 percent organically produced raw or processed foods.
- *Organic*   Products with 95 to 100 percent organic ingredients can use this label. Up to 5 percent of the food can come from non-organic foods approved on a national list.
- *Made with organic [specific ingredients]*   Products that contain 50 to 95 percent organic ingredients can use this label and must list up to three organic ingredients on the principal display panel. For example, if a granola is labeled cereal "made with organic oats, rice and raisins," it means that these three ingredients are organic, but other ingredients in the product are not.
- *No label, but the product contains some organic ingredients*   A food product that contains up to 50 percent organic ingredients may list the specifically grown ingredients within the ingredients section on the food label. As an example, a granola bar with organic raisins but no other organic ingredients can list organic raisins as one of the ingredients on the label.

The National Organic Program within the USDA is charged with the responsibility to oversee and monitor farms that produce organic food.

FAQS about organic foods

Although more and more organic food products arrive every day on produce and grocery shelves and in meat sections of many supermarkets, there is still some confusion about the foods themselves. On its website, *www.ams.usda.gov/nop*, The National Organic Program provides answers to many of the questions that have been asked about these foods since 1990. Here is a small sampling:

How is organic produce certified?

Farmers must grow produce for three years without the application of synthetic pesticides or chemicals. The farm, its equipment, and any processing facilities are inspected by an independent agency unaffiliated with the grower, the processor or the vendor, and the farm is issued a certificate from that agency certifying the farm's produce as "organic."

Can meat be certified "organic"?

Livestock can be certified "organic" if it has been raised on organic feedstuffs (grains and other products grown under certified organic conditions) for at least a year and are given sufficient time for grazing on pasturelands as opposed to complete confinement.

Why is organic produce more expensive than the other kind?

Organic produce, since it is grown without synthetic pesticides or chemicals, is more labor-intensive. Organic crop yields are often not as high as those grown under non-organic conditions, and fewer farmers (only about 4%) use organic methods and sustainable agriculture practices; therefore the price of organically grown produce reflects the greater demands placed on the grower. Most people will notice that the price of organic foods has dropped over the last few years as they have gained popularity.

**Is organically grown produce healthier
than other produce?**

Certified organic produce is not essentially healthier than produce
that has been grown under non-organic conditions—the nutritional
content of a particular vegetable doesn't change. But the lack of synthetic pesticidal residues on organically grown produce definitely
makes for a safer product.

THE CONTROVERSY OVER GENETICALLY
MODIFIED (GM) FOODS

Organic foods are at the opposite end of the spectrum from foods that
have been genetically modified (GM, also referred to as GE, or genetically engineered). My colleagues and I continue to debate the pros and cons
of GM foods and will do so for a long time to come.

The most compelling claim for GM foods is that they can help feed the
world and bring an end to hunger. If we can increase crop production, wipe
out diseases such as blindness and anemia in developing countries, increase
the protein content of various foods to decrease malnutrition in poorer nations, and increase the shelf life of perishable foods, among other benefits,
we will have improved and extended the lives of countless millions. By doing
so, its proponents claim, GM foods will be a powerful, humanitarian way for
science to serve social policy.

To buttress these claims, GM scientists say that GM foods are just like
natural foods; they are simply an extension of traditional crossbreeding.

Opponents of GM foods believe that we are playing God and manipulat-
ing the balance of nature—and that the consequences could be devastating.
GM foods, they say, are not natural; otherwise seed producers wouldn't take
out patents on the seeds. Increasing and even improving the food supply
alone cannot eliminate hunger; it's poverty, wars, and infrastructure that
prevent nations from buying food and distributing it.

I have not reached a definitive conclusion about GM foods. Right now there is much that we don't know or understand about how these foods will affect our lives. The issues are exceptionally complex, and there are still so many unresolved scientific, social, and ethical questions that it would be irresponsible to make a blanket judgment right now.

But I am strongly in favor of using greater caution when it comes to experimenting with GM foods. For me, the problem with arguments in favor of them is that they are supported primarily by huge industries—the giant chemical and seed companies and the universities whose scientific facilities are funded by these industries. Certainly, there are many scientists and some corporations interested in the humanitarian work of eliminating blindness and other health problems with GM foods. But a more pressing reason is that corporations have invested huge sums of money in GM foods, and they want a high yield on those investments, soon. These are economic, not humanitarian, reasons.

What's in a name?

The crossbreeding of different species has been practiced for millennia without the need for a new terminology beyond the familiar word *hybrid* and its variations. Twentieth- and twenty-first-century science has spawned, so to speak, a new set of terms to describe the processes and products of the genetic revolution. As applied to food and nutrition, two of these, and their acronyms, are genetic modification (GM) and genetic engineering (GE), which describe the same process.

How is food genetically engineered?

Genetic engineering is a laboratory technique that can be considered a form of artificial insemination. One gene or, more often, a set of several genes is removed from the DNA of an organism (the donor cell), transported via a carrier (sometimes bacteria or a virus), and inserted into the DNA of another organism (the recipient cell). Because there is currently no way to insert a gene into a predetermined location, the insertion can be haphazard. Unlike human artificial insemination, in GE the DNA of one species is being crossed with that of a completely different species, a procedure that is also described as crossing the species barrier. If the genetic engineering works, the recipient organism then takes on the new desired trait from the new gene.

An example of the kinds of improvement GM scientists are aiming for can be seen in the modification of tomatoes. Tomatoes do not survive in cold weather. Fish such as flounder have a high resistance to cold. Scientists have identified the cold-resistant gene in flounder and have injected it into tomatoes, which allows the GE tomatoes to have a longer growing season.

A brief look at the long history of crossbreeding

Animals and crops have been crossbred for food production ever since human beings invented agriculture and began to domesticate animals. Our ancestors crossbred crops and livestock to develop the varieties that were resistant to cold or to heat, foods that would not be demolished by pests, foods that tasted and looked better. This crossbreeding enhanced diversity in crops and animals instead of diminishing it.

Starting about 20 years ago, scientists began to experiment with the genetic modification of certain foods. By 1997, a wide variety of GM foods (all unlabeled) entered the marketplace. The manufacturers claim the products are perfectly safe but still don't want the words *GE ingredients* to appear on the nutrition facts label because they think the public will be alarmed, and they may be right. As of this writing, GE labeling is not required by either the FDA or the USDA. However, there are a number of food producers who are voluntarily labeling their products as being *free* of GM ingredients. So, if you want to avoid GE foods, your best bet is to eat "certified organic" foods, because by law they cannot contain genetically engineered ingredients.

Corn and soybeans are currently the most prevalent GE foods because they are used in such a wide range of products: margarine, chocolate, bread, soda, spaghetti sauce, and potato chips, to name just a few. GE corn and soybeans are also grown for animal feed and used in the United States and worldwide. This means that animals all over the world are eating fodder whose long-term effects are still unknown.

The case for golden rice

The specific instance of golden rice is a favorable example of GE. The research to develop transgenic rice was conducted in the early 1990s by German and Swiss universities and funded by the Rockefeller Foundation and Swiss governmental and European Union programs. The scientists involved in this ambitious project have said repeatedly that once the rice proves to be viable and beneficial, it will be freely distributed and that no patents will hinder access to it by farmers in developing nations.

The research did succeed in developing rice plants that synthesize more beta-carotene (a precursor to vitamin A) in the endosperm of the kernel. Vitamin A deficiency is the leading cause of blindness in the world. While beta-carotene is contained naturally in the whole grain of non-GM rice, once that rice is milled the beta-carotene is lost. In this new variety of GM rice, the beta-carotene is present in the endosperm, which remains after milling, so the grain is a rich supply of beta-carotene and could be of enormous benefit in countries where unrefined brown rice is not eaten. Because of patent issues, golden rice has not yet been released for agricultural use.

We do not know the long-term impact of these crops on the environment over the next decades. But we do know that there is genuine humanitarian intention behind the development of golden rice, and if it is successful, it could significantly help to reduce blindness in developing countries.

Health and environmental concerns about GE foods

Biotech food is wracked by controversy, and not just in the United States. Japan, Australia, and the European Union, among others, require labeling of GE foods. Worldwide, there is a large and vocal opposition of scientists, informed consumers, environmentalists, and other activists. Each group has its own agenda, and each is interested in raising the consciousness of people in general, food producers and purveyors, and governmental agencies in

The case for monarch butterflies (and against Bt corn)

The case for monarch butterflies is one against GE foods. In a Cornell University study published in *Nature,* researchers noted that GM corn has genes from the bacterium Bacillus thuringiensis (Bt), an insecticide, spliced into the plant genes. These hybrids are very effective against the European corn borer, a major corn pest that is destroyed by the plant's toxic tissue.

Unlike many pesticides, the Bt corn has been shown to have no effect on many "nontarget" organisms—pollinators, such as honeybees, or beneficial predators of pests, such as ladybugs. But the Bt-modified corn produces pollen that also contains Bt. When the pollen is dispersed by the wind, it lands on other plants, including milkweed, which is the exclusive food of monarch caterpillars and is commonly found around cornfields.

In laboratory tests, a group of monarch caterpillars was fed milkweed leaves dusted with so-called "transformed" pollen from a Bt corn hybrid. These caterpillars ate less, grew more slowly, and suffered a higher mortality rate—nearly half of them died. There were also two control groups of monarch caterpillars in the study: one was fed leaves dusted with non-transformed corn pollen, and the other was fed leaves without any corn pollen at all. All of the caterpillars in the two control groups survived the study.

It was found that the Bt in the transformed pollen goes into the caterpillar's intestine, where it binds to specific sites. When the toxin binds, the intestine wall changes from a protective layer to an open sieve, so that pathogens usually kept within the intestine and excreted are released into the insect's body. The caterpillar quickly sickens and dies. Monarch caterpillars feed on milkweed during the period when corn is shedding pollen, which may account for their exposure to Bt pollen.

The Cornell report became a cause célèbre, triggering accusations on all sides of the GE issue and an acceleration of the ongoing reevaluation of GE crops. Although the EPA, in September 2000, issued a preliminary report saying that biotech corn was not likely to pose a threat to monarchs, more studies in the wild are underway.

particular to the potential perils of an unchecked spread of GE seeds and foods. Here are some of their concerns:

- The laboratory technique of removing a gene from an organism is easily accomplished, but transferring it to a new organism cannot be achieved with precision. This random placement could have a negative effect on other genes within the recipient organism and may possibly cause harmful genetic mutations down the road in plants, animals, or humans.
- Scientists are intentionally engineering seeds that all contain the same genetic makeup to produce crops that are identical. If a virus, fungus, or pest (a superbug) should develop that is capable of destroying plants with specific genetic characteristics, entire crops could be destroyed, instead of only part of the crop.
- Insects, birds, and wind can transport GE seeds and pollen to new locations. Should this happen on a large scale, our entire food supply would be at risk of contamination and vulnerable to any of the problems that apply to GE products.
- No long-term, impartial testing has been conducted on the effects of consuming GE foods or growing with GE seeds. Testing standards have not been determined for many processed foods, and the sheer quantity of genes that are being injected into plants makes their detection at any stage questionable.
- GE foods could potentially cause new and severe allergic reactions.
- Biotech foods have been engineered to have a longer shelf life. Although a food might appear "fresh," the nutritional value might be substantially reduced over time.

The major concern for ecologists and environmentalists is the potential for damage and destruction of the environment. People voicing these doubts have been called alarmists by GE corporations and by our government, which has held that genetically engineered foods are safe for people, safe for the environment.

According to Greenpeace, by 2000, the world had lost 95 percent of the genetic diversity that existed in agriculture only 100 years earlier. The chance that we could lose that last 5 percent through the spread, intentional or otherwise, of genetically engineered seeds and crops is what haunts those of us who question the wisdom of more genetic engineering without sound, scientific, impartial testing of all the potential effects of this new, thrilling, frightening science.

WHERE ARE WE NOW? WHERE DO WE GO FROM HERE?

By the time most of the food you eat arrives on your table, it has been through three basic and interdependent steps: production, processing, and transportation. Primarily because of technological advances, each of these steps, separately and together, has undergone radical transformation in the last fifty years.

What's better?

Many of the changes in our food supply have been beneficial, not just in America, but throughout the world. For instance, it is now possible to grow and ship enough food to feed every person in every nation. Although millions still go hungry due to environmental factors, poor infrastructure, human corruption, and unspeakable poverty, there would still be sufficient food for them if those nations with overstocks were allowed to deliver food to the people who need it.

In the United States and many other developed nations, government has worked with food producers and processors to establish health and safety standards and to provide oversight. This means that almost all of the food we eat and much of the water we drink is safe and dependable.

There have been extensive changes for the better in the preservation and storage of foods. Techniques for freezing and canning have improved. Irradiation, in which foods are exposed to radiant energy as a means of extending shelf life, have been thoroughly tested by the FDA and approved as safe for meats, fruits, and other foods. Altered atmosphere storage facilities have made it possible to eat a number of fresh fruits and vegetables almost year round.

For Americans, one of the most pleasurable culinary improvements in the last fifty years is the adoption of formerly foreign foods. Fruits and vegetables once considered exotic we now take for granted. Although many are still imported, others have been so warmly embraced that they are grown and produced here.

Altered atmosphere storage

In 1940, Cornell University pioneered altered atmosphere (AA, originally called controlled atmosphere, or CA) storage, the technology that is used to extend the shelf life of some fruits and vegetables. Before then, apples could be stored for four months, at most, and by the end of that period they were mushy and beginning to decay. With AA, onions can be stored for up to five months, and apples can be stored for up to ten months.

AA storage chambers are sealed rooms designed to create the proper temperature, humidity, and air composition to maintain the quality of produce for long periods of time. Newly harvested fruits are packed in special containers and placed in the refrigerated rooms, which are kept at 30° to 31° F, with a relative humidity of 90 to 95 percent. The oxygen supply is then lowered to about 5 percent and the carbon dioxide concentration increased, which allows the fruit to enter a "vegetative" state that inhibits ripening. The rooms can be opened at any time from three to ten months after they are sealed, and the fruit tastes almost as fresh and flavorful as the day it was stored.

AA began with apples, but pears, grapes, bananas, and onions have been added to the list, and they are now available almost year-round.

What's worse?

Other changes in our food supply have been less positive, and their conse-quences have created questions and difficult choices for us now and in the future.

The disappearance of the local family farm, often referred to as the back-bone of our nation, is a matter of deep concern. These are the farms that produce the freshest, tastiest, healthiest food that we put on the table. And when the farms are organic as well, they protect and improve the environ-ment. With the growing public interest in organic foods and the support of some governmental agencies and independent farmers' groups, it is possible that more small farmers will turn toward organic farming, more farms will be started, and the trend will be reversed—but not quickly.

GE foods, which I've already discussed in this chapter, may have the most long-range effects of any changes made in our food supply during the last fifty years. One day, there are no biotech foods; the next, they are all around us, and we don't know what they are. The questions raised in this chapter, and others, are now being asked not just by scientists and consumer groups but by a public uneasy with the idea of genetic manipulation. There is more to come.

FOOD ADDITIVES

Since there are currently more than 10,000 food additives in use, it would be foolhardy of me to attempt to name and explain all but a few of them.

The first additives were food preservatives, such as salt, vinegar, and sugar. Today, preservatives and other additives, whether natural or man-made, are used to preserve, sweeten, enhance flavor, and improve the tex-ture and color of foods. Some additives are beneficial, as is the case when vitamins and minerals are added to enrich staple foods such as grains, milk, soy products, juices, and others. Most additives are safe; some are not so safe.

Here is a very brief look at some of the additives you will encounter as you peruse the thousands of food products on supermarket shelves:

- Nitrate and nitrite are used as preservatives in smoked fish, ham, bacon, sausage, and other processed meats, particularly meats found at the deli counter. It is well known that sodium nitrite can be converted to nitrous acid in the human body and that nitrous acid has been shown to increase rates of cancer in animals. Nevertheless, these preservatives are still used in almost every commercially produced ham, salami, sausage, bologna, etc., that you can buy, with very few preservative-free alternatives. Fortunately, these foods must be labeled. Also fortunately, there are more and more butchers who make their own preservative-free sausages (including chicken sausages), but unless you have access to them, your best bet is to eat foods that contain nitrate no more than once or twice a week.
- Antioxidants are often used as preservatives in fatty foods to prevent spoilage. BHT (butylated hydroxytoluene) and BHA (butylated hydroxyanisole) are the two most widely used. Although tests on both additives have produced a host of alarming results, they are added to thousands of processed foods. Countries such as Sweden, Romania, Australia, and Great Britain have severely restricted their use; by contrast, in the United States their use has increased. Vitamin E is another antioxidant that is sometimes added to oils and is perfectly safe and also healthy.
- Monosodium glutamate (MSG), a flavor enhancer, is still pervasive in imported Asian foods. Aside from its aftertaste, some people are sensitive to MSG, which is thought to cause headaches after eating it.
- Emulsifiers and stabilizers such as lecithin, guar gum, and carrageenin are used to prevent foods such as peanut butter from separating. These additives seem to be very safe.

We have come a long way in the past hundred years in terms of production, distribution, and storage of food. In America today, more food is available to more people, and in greater variety, than ever before. Organic food is making a comeback and giving us even more options. I believe that most of these advances are for the better, but not, in my view, all for the better. Our food now is more processed and contains greater numbers of additives, and most of us have no idea under what conditions the food was grown.

Regarding genetic modification, as a scientist myself, I believe that if we could eradicate blindness by adding beta-carotene to rice—without imperiling the environment—it *would* be a miracle, and I would applaud it. But as a scientist working in nutrition, I also feel we must be aware of what we're eating and careful of how far and how fast we go in changing our food supply. In my own family, we try to stay with whole foods and fresh produce, and whenever possible, we support our local farmers.

In the larger worlds of academia, industry, and governments, prudence, rigorous scientific testing, and a consideration of long-range consequences should be the basis of any decisions about developing and producing new foods.

Strong Women Eat Well

The Recipes

❖

One of the most rewarding parts of writing this book has been working on the recipes with Judy Knipe, my collaborator. I've never considered myself a cook. Although I like to make meals for company and for the family, the ingredients I use and my methods of preparation are pretty basic. What I've always wanted is a little more pizzazz in my cooking, and that's what Judy has provided.

A colleague of mine who knows her well told me that much of what she had learned about good food she learned from Judy. After working with Judy on the recipes, I now know what she means. My cooking really improved while we were writing this book—much to the delight of my husband and kids—because I agreed to test most of the recipes. By now, a number of them are staples in our weekly meals, and my family and dinner guests really appreciate the changes in my culinary repertoire.

Before Judy and I even talked about the recipes, we discussed my ideas and my philosophy of good eating. My approach to nutrition—my message—is that optimal health and pleasure in eating are best achieved through a varied diet of mostly whole foods. But I also believe that there is room for almost any kind of food. These are the guidelines I gave Judy:

- Use whole foods.
- Experiment with foods that people may find unfamiliar so that they can add variety to their diets.
- Use a lot of whole grains to increase fiber.
- Use fruits and vegetables in a variety of recipes.
- Be sure to have a number of recipes using calcium-rich foods.
- Develop recipes with soy foods.
- Create recipes that can be recycled as delicious leftovers that can be used in other dishes.
- Develop recipes that can be adapted easily to different tastes.
- Create recipes with interesting textures and contrasting colors and flavors.

Some of these recipes are quite adventurous, with wonderful fusions of tastes that I had not experienced before. Although most of the ingredients are whole foods, healthy foods, some of the recipes do include butter or cream and salt. I think that these foods are fine in moderation, and they add so much pleasure to the meal that they deserve their place at the table.

If you are on a weight control program, you will need to limit the amount of fat in your diet. It's equally important for *everyone* to control portion sizes, as well. If you want more information about nutrition and exercise for long-term weight control, I hope you will read my book, *Strong Women Stay Slim*, which many people have found very helpful.

And now, on to the recipes. I hope you'll try them, enjoy them, and use them often.

RECIPE LIST

Fish

Poultry

Grains

Vegetables

Desserts

Beverages

To the readers of *Strong Women Stay Slim*

Strong Women Eat Well is not a weight-loss book. Instead, I wrote it to give you the means for achieving a healthy diet of delicious, whole foods—a diet based on the most recent scientific information about good nutrition and good health.

You will notice that the yields in recipes that follow are in a somewhat different format from those in *Strong Women Stay Slim*. The yields here are expressed simply as the number of servings in each recipe, not how many portions each serving contains (one vegetable portion, two grain portions, and so on). I did this primarily because I wanted the readers of this book to focus on the entire diet, on whole foods, and on the great pleasure to be had in eating them rather than being distracted by numbers.

However, if you have been following the program in *Strong Women Stay Slim,* you will easily be able to look at a recipe and see how many portions of each food group it contains and how it fits into your overall food plan. Many of the recipes have options that will allow you to adapt them for your own weight control needs.

It is very important for you to maintain a healthy body weight. By using the nutritional information in *Strong Women Eat Well* and the weight-loss program in *Strong Women Stay Slim,* you will unite these goals—as eating well and staying slim go hand in hand.

PRESERVED LEMONS

❖

Makes 2 pints

I hope this will be the first recipe you make from the book. I was inspired to add this recipe when a dear friend served me a delicious roast chicken rubbed with preserved lemon. He told me how versatile the lemons are, and he was right.

Although you'll spend only minutes preparing the lemons, it takes six weeks for them to reach their perfect pickled preservation. And once you begin cooking with them, you will want to have them on hand always. Often I simply throw them into a tossed salad. Recipes that call for the lemons are Green Sauce (page 192); Poached Salmon (page 207); Broiled Salmon Fillet (page 206); Tuna Salad with Preserved Lemon (page 209); Chicken Breasts with Squash, Tomatoes, and Preserved Lemon (page 211); and Brown Rice Salad with Green Vegetables (page 217). I know you'll find many other uses for this wonderful condiment.

10 or 11 lemons
kosher salt

Before you prepare the lemons, sterilize two 1-pint canning jars (wide-mouthed is best). This is very easy to do. Simply place the jars on a rack in a large pan and add enough boiling water to fill and cover them. Boil for 5 minutes, adding the caps during the last minute. Remove the jars and let them drain and cool upside down on a rack.

Wash the lemons, and cut off the tips of the stem ends. Cut 7 or 8 of the lemons, depending on their size, into lengthwise quarters, remove the seeds with the tip of a sharp knife, and gently squeeze a little of the juice from each quarter into a measuring cup or another spouted vessel. Make a small nick in the center of each cut edge and flatten out the lemon quarters. Pour a small mound of kosher salt on a plate or piece of wax paper, and rub salt all over the lemons. Press them into the jars as you go along, leaving as little space as possible between each piece. Fill the jars with lemons, leaving about ½ inch of headroom at the top. Pour in the reserved juice, then juice as many of the other lemons as you need to completely cover the lemon quarters. Seal the jars.

Leave the lemons out at room temperature for one week, turning the jars upside-down once a day to distribute the brine equally among all the pieces. Refrigerate for another five weeks. Use as directed.

YOGURT SAUCE WITH GINGER AND ONION

❖

Makes a scant 2 cups

Serve the sauce with lentils or whole grains such as brown rice, couscous, or whole wheatberries.

2 teaspoons safflower or canola oil
1 or 2 cloves garlic, peeled and minced
1-inch chunk fresh ginger, peeled and minced
pinch cayenne pepper
½ cup finely chopped red or Vidalia onion
1½ cups plain low-fat yogurt
2 tablespoons chopped fresh coriander
2 tablespoons chopped fresh mint

Heat the oil in a small skillet or saucepan over a moderate flame, add the garlic and ginger, and sauté just until the garlic is a little softened, 1 or 2 minutes. Scrape the mixture into a bowl and add the remaining ingredients. Serve at room temperature or cold.

GREEN SAUCE

❖

Makes a generous ½ cup

There are many versions of green sauce used throughout the Mediterranean as an accompaniment to fish, boiled meats, and steamed vegetables, such as steamed cauliflower, or as a spread on bread. Crisp, curly parsley
is easy to chop in the food processor and tastes very good in this recipe. The
preserved lemon is an optional ingredient, but it adds sparkle to the finished
sauce. A small amount of this sauce carries a lot of flavor, so don't slather it on.

  2 garlic cloves, peeled
  2 cups packed, curly parsley leaves
  1 quarter Preserved Lemon (page 190), rinsed, pulp
     discarded, and quartered (optional)
  1 tablespoon tiny capers
  1 tablespoon red wine vinegar
  1 tablespoon fresh lemon juice
  ½ cup extra-virgin olive oil

With the motor of the processor running, drop the garlic through the feed
tube and chop it. Add the parsley and process until it is very finely chopped.
Add the lemon rind and process until chopped. Add the capers, vinegar,
lemon juice, and olive oil and process until the capers are chopped and
the sauce is well mixed. Keeps for two days, tightly covered, in the refrigerator.

MARINARA SAUCE

❖

Makes 3 to 3½ cups

The vegetables for this fresh-tasting sauce can be chopped in a moment
with a food processor. After that the sauce cooks for about 20 minutes and
is ready to serve over pasta or use in any recipe calling for a tomato sauce.

1 tablespoon extra-virgin olive oil
1 or 2 cloves garlic, peeled and minced
1 medium onion, peeled and minced
1 small carrot, chopped
1 celery stalk, trimmed and chopped
pinch red pepper flakes (optional)
1 28-ounce can whole tomatoes (preferably organic),
 pulsed several times in food processor
salt
freshly ground black pepper

Place a heavy 2-quart saucepan over moderate to low heat, add the oil, garlic, onions, carrots, celery, and red pepper flakes, if using, and sauté for 10
minutes, stirring often. Add tomatoes and salt and pepper to taste and bring
to a simmer. Simmer gently for 10 minutes and taste for seasoning. Store in
refrigerator for two days or freeze for up to three months.

Tuna and Olive Sauce for Pasta

Add one 6-ounce can of tuna fish packed in olive oil, drained, ½ cup oil-
cured black olives (Kalamata or Gaeta), pitted, and 3 or 4 tablespoons
chopped flat parsley to the finished sauce and cook just until hot. Enough for
12 to 16 ounces of pasta.

YOGURT WITH GARLIC
AND CUCUMBER

❖

Makes 2½ to 3 cups

I like this condiment as an accompaniment to grains or poached or broiled salmon. It's also a welcome addition to a buffet table. European or Kirby cucumbers are preferable because their skins are not waxed and they need not be seeded. However, if neither of these is available, use regular cucumbers, peeled, halved, and seeded.

    2 cloves garlic, peeled and minced
    2 teaspoons fruity extra-virgin olive oil
    1½ cups plain low-fat yogurt
    1 to 1½ cups diced unpeeled European or Kirby cucumber
    salt and freshly ground black pepper to taste
    3 to 4 tablespoons chopped fresh mint or basil or snipped
        fresh dill

Combine all the ingredients in a bowl and mix well. Cover and let stand for an hour. Serve cold or at room temperature.

GRAPEFRUIT SALSA

❖

Makes about 1 cup

You'll need a really sharp paring knife for this recipe. The plain salsa is wonderful with grilled or broiled fish or poultry or hot sausages. The variation with avocado is sublime.

1 grapefruit
fresh hot pepper to taste, stemmed, cored, and minced
¼ cup chopped red onion
2 teaspoons lime juice
1 tablespoon chopped fresh coriander
small pinch salt

Hold the fruit over a bowl to catch the juices, then, with a sharp paring knife, cut off the rind and pith, exposing the flesh. Keeping the knife close to the membrane, cut down along the side of one segment to the core. Free the segment by cutting along the membrane on the other side. Let the segments drop into the bowl as you cut them. When you are done, you will have a handful of membranes; with very little juicy flesh attached. If you want a really liquid salsa, squeeze the juice into the bowl and discard the membranes; otherwise, just squeeze the juice into a glass and drink it yourself as a special treat.

The kind and amount of fresh hot pepper you use is up to you. Add it with the onion, lime juice, coriander, and salt. Serve cold or at room temperature.

Grapefruit Salsa with Avocado

Peel and pit ½ Hass avocado, cut into ½-inch dice, and stir into the grapefruit salsa. Serve in small bowls or over greens as a first course.

CREAM OF TOMATO SOUP

❖

Serves 4 to 6

Flavorful canned tomatoes are the key to the success of this soup, which can be made in about 35 minutes and which freezes very well.

1 tablespoon butter
1 medium onion, peeled, quartered, and sliced
1 28-ounce can plum tomatoes (preferably organic)
2 tablespoons tomato paste
2 cups chicken stock or canned chicken broth
1 tablespoon brown sugar
1 bay leaf
pinch of cayenne or dried hot pepper flakes (optional)
pinch allspice
2 whole cloves or a pinch ground cloves
salt
freshly ground black pepper
1 cup half-and-half

Melt the butter over medium heat in a heavy saucepan, add the onion, and sauté, covered, until translucent, 3 or 4 minutes. Add the tomatoes with their juices, the tomato paste, chicken stock, brown sugar, bay leaf, cayenne (if desired), allspice, cloves, and salt and pepper to taste. Bring to a boil, lower the heat, and simmer, covered, for 20 minutes.

Remove the bay leaf and strain the soup over a bowl. Puree the solids in a blender or food processor, adding some of the strained liquid as needed. Rinse the saucepan. Return the liquid and puree to the saucepan (strain the puree through a fine-mesh sieve if you wish), add the half-and-half, and bring the soup to a simmer. Cook for 5 minutes and taste for seasonings.

Cream of Tomato Soup Provençal

The extra garlic, orange zest, and saffron add a subtle Provençal touch. Don't omit the cayenne for this recipe.

Substitute olive oil for the butter and sauté 2 or 3 cloves chopped garlic with the onion. Add 3 or 4 long strips orange zest and a large pinch of saffron threads with the tomatoes and cook as directed. Puree the zest with the tomatoes, and continue with the recipe, reducing the half-and-half to ½ cup.

HONEY MUSTARD–
BALSAMIC VINEGAR GLAZE

❖

I brush this mixture on poultry, salmon fillet, or pork tenderloin before roasting or broiling. Use an amount that is appropriate for the food you are cooking.

1 part mild honey, such as alfalfa or clover
1 part Dijon mustard
1 part balsamic vinegar

Place all the ingredients in a small bowl and whisk to combine.

CARROT SOUP WITH FRESH GINGER

❖

Serves 5 or 6

The cream is not absolutely necessary, but it adds a luxurious flavor and texture. This is a terrific make-ahead soup, very good served cold, and it freezes well for two or three months.

2 small onions or 1 medium onion, peeled, halved, and sliced
2 to 3 tablespoons unsalted butter
1½ pounds carrots, peeled and cut into medium chunks
1½ quarts chicken stock or canned chicken broth
½ teaspoon ground coriander
salt
freshly ground pepper
1 or 2 tablespoons fresh ginger, peeled and grated
½ cup half-and-half (optional)

Garnish

plain low-fat or nonfat yogurt
chopped fresh coriander or chives

In a medium saucepan over moderate heat, sauté the onion in the butter for 3 to 4 minutes, or until translucent. Add the carrots, chicken stock, ground coriander, and salt and pepper to taste, and bring to a boil. Cover the pan, lower the heat, and cook gently for about 25 minutes, or until the carrots are very tender. Puree the soup in batches in a food processor or blender, and return to the pan. (If you are a truly compulsive cook, you might want to force the carrot puree through a fine mesh sieve to make an even silkier puree, but the soup will taste just fine if you omit this step.) Add grated fresh ginger to taste and the half-and-half, if desired, and adjust the seasonings.

Serve the soup hot, warm, or cold, garnished with a spoonful of yogurt and chopped coriander or chives.

FISH AND CORN CHOWDER

❖

Serves 4 to 6

On a cold fall day, there's nothing more comforting than a fish and corn
chowder—and nothing easier, either.

1 tablespoon olive oil
1 cup chopped onion
12 ounces potatoes, peeled and cut into ½-inch dice
1 bay leaf
2 cups fish stock or chicken stock or canned chicken broth,
    or a combination
salt
freshly ground pepper
1½ pounds firm fish fillets, such as scrod,
    cut into large chunks
2 cups corn kernels (fresh or frozen)
2 cups milk
1 tablespoon unsalted butter

Heat the olive oil in a heavy 4-quart saucepan, add the onion and potatoes,
and sauté over moderate heat for 10 minutes or until the onion is translucent
and the potatoes have begun to take on color. Add the bay leaf, stock, and
salt and pepper to taste. Bring to a simmer and cook slowly until the potatoes
are tender, about 10 minutes. Add the fish, corn, and milk, and return to a
simmer. Cook another few minutes, just until the fish is opaque. Do not boil.
Adjust the seasoning, add the butter, and allow it to melt. Remove the bay
leaf before serving.

Mushroom Soup

❖

Serves 6 to 8

This is a rich, thick, earthy soup whose intense flavor comes courtesy of dried porcini mushrooms. The flavor improves if the soup is made a day before serving it. Because its color is an uncompromising grayish-brown, be sure to sprinkle each serving with chopped parsley, chives, or scallion tops.

1 ounce dried porcini mushrooms (available at gourmet food shops, or see Resources, page 257)

2½ cups water

2 tablespoons unsalted butter

1 medium onion, peeled, quartered, and sliced

1 medium leek, ends and green leaves trimmed, split, washed, and sliced

2 cloves garlic, peeled and sliced

2 carrots, peeled and sliced

1½ pounds white mushrooms, stem ends trimmed and sliced

4 cups chicken stock or canned chicken broth

salt

freshly ground pepper

1 cup half-and-half

freshly grated nutmeg

chopped parsley or sliced chives or scallion tops

In a small saucepan, combine the dried porcini and the water and bring to a boil over high heat. Cover the pan, reduce the heat to low, and simmer the mushrooms for 15 minutes. Drain, reserving the liquid and the mushrooms separately. Rinse off the mushrooms under running water, rubbing them with your fingers to dislodge any residual sand lurking in the folds. Strain the cooking liquid through a coffee filter or a sieve lined with a dampened paper towel. Reserve.

In a medium saucepan, melt the butter over moderate heat, add the onion, leek, garlic, and carrots, and cook for about 5 minutes, stirring, or until the onion is translucent. Add the white mushrooms and cook, stirring occasionally, for 5 minutes. Add the chicken stock, reserved porcini mushrooms, strained mushroom broth, and salt and pepper to taste. Bring to a simmer and cook, partially covered, for about 30 minutes.

Strain the soup into a bowl, transferring the solids to a food processor, and puree the solids, adding a ladle or two of the broth and scraping down the sides of the bowl as needed. Return the liquid and puree to the saucepan and reheat. Add the half-and-half and a light grating of nutmeg and taste for seasoning. Cook for 3 or 4 minutes longer. Stir well from the bottom when ladling out the soup. Serve hot, sprinkled with chopped parsley, sliced chives, or scallion tops. Store up to three days in refrigerator, tightly covered, and up to two months in freezer.

COLD SPELT AND LENTIL SOUP
WITH HERBS AND CRISP VEGETABLES

❖

Serves 4 to 6

Soft, chewy, crunchy—three textures at work in a tart, faintly lemony soup. It takes longer to read the recipe than it does to make it. This is a festive soup, which you can make well ahead of time.

Soup

½ cup spelt (available at health-food stores)
½ cup brown or green lentils
salt
1½ cups organic low-fat or no-fat yogurt
grated zest of ½ lemon
1 tablespoon fresh lemon juice
freshly ground black pepper

Herbs and Greens (use 2 or 3)

1 cup chopped or finely sliced mint, flat parsley, dill,
  coriander, basil, scallion tops, watercress leaves, young
  mustard greens, spinach, or arugula

*Raw Vegetables (¾ cup per serving; choose 3 to 5 vegetables,
with flavor, color, texture, and availability as a guide; be
sure to use tomatoes, available year-round)*

chopped radishes; red or Vidalia onion; scallions; Kirby or
  European seedless cucumbers; red, green, and yellow bell
  peppers; fennel; finely chopped jalapeño pepper; halved
  grape or cherry tomatoes

Combine the spelt and 1 quart of water in a medium saucepan and bring to
a boil over high heat. Reduce the heat, cover the pan, and simmer for 35 to
40 minutes, or until the spelt is partially cooked. Add the lentils and salt to
taste and return to a boil. Reduce the heat, cover the pot, and simmer until
the lentils and grain are tender, 30 to 40 minutes, depending on the type and
age of the lentils. Remove from the heat, then cool and chill the soup.

Add the yogurt, lemon zest, and lemon juice to the soup and stir until
well blended. Taste for seasoning (don't neglect the black pepper). Chill until
serving time.

No more than 3 hours before serving the soup, chop the herbs and cut up
the raw vegetables and store separately, well covered, in the refrigerator. To
serve, ladle the soup into bowls, sprinkle liberally with the chopped herbs,
and pass a bowl with the vegetables separately.

Storage: Leftover soup can be stored, tightly covered, in the refrigerator for
three or four days. Herbs and vegetables should be prepared within a few
hours of serving time to preserve their freshness and nutritional values.

Asparagus and Ham Frittata

❖

Each frittata serves 2

Traditionally, frittatas are baked until set in a moderate oven, but I must admit that often I take the path of least resistance and simply cover the skillet and cook the eggs on top of the stove. The first two frittatas here are baked, the second two are stovetop recipes.

> ¾ to 1 pound asparagus
> salt
> 2 teaspoons butter
> 2 ounces baked or boiled ham, diced
> 3 eggs
> freshly ground white pepper

Preheat the oven to 350° F.

Cut off the asparagus tips and set aside. Trim off and discard the woody ends. Cut the spears in ¾-inch lengths and place in a small nonstick skillet. Add water to cover, salt to taste, and bring to a boil. Cook for 1 minute, add the asparagus tips, and cook 1 minute longer. Drain and reserve asparagus in the sieve. Melt the butter in the skillet over moderate heat, add the ham, and fry for 2 minutes, stirring until it just begins to color. Add the asparagus and cook until heated. Beat the eggs, add salt and pepper to taste, and pour over the ham and asparagus. Cook just until the bottom is set, about 1 minute, then bake for 10 to 12 minutes, or until the top is just set. Slide out of the pan onto a serving plate and allow to cool for 5 to 8 minutes before serving.

Asparagus and Oyster Mushroom Frittata

Substitute 1 to 2 cups of the asparagus and oyster mushroom version of Stir-Fried Green Vegetables and Mushrooms (page 228). Bake at 350° F until set.

ROASTED VEGETABLE FRITTATA

❖

2 teaspoons olive oil
¾ to 1 cup roasted or grilled vegetables,
   cut into ½- to 1-inch pieces
3 eggs
salt
freshly ground pepper
2 or 3 tablespoons grated Jack or cheddar cheese

Heat the oil in a small skillet, preferably nonstick, over moderate heat. Add the roasted vegetables and cook until hot. Beat the eggs with salt and pepper to taste and pour over the vegetables. Sprinkle with the cheese. Lower the heat, cover, and cook on top of stove, just until the omelet is set, but still soft. Transfer to a plate and cool for 8 to 10 minutes before eating. Nice with a salad and whole-grain toast.

PEPPER AND ONION FRITTATA

❖

2 teaspoons olive oil
1 medium red or green bell pepper, cored, seeded,
   and cut into ½-inch strips
1 medium onion, peeled, halved, and sliced
3 eggs
salt
freshly ground black pepper
chopped parsley

Heat the oil in a well-oiled cast-iron or small nonstick skillet over a moderate flame. Add the pepper and onion and cook, stirring often, until the vegetables are soft and just beginning to brown. Beat the eggs with salt and pepper to taste, beat in the parsley, and pour over the vegetables. Lower the heat, cover, and cook on top of stove, just until the omelet is set, but still soft. Transfer to a plate and cool for 8 to 10 minutes before eating.

SPINACH AND CHEDDAR EGG SUPPER

❖

Serves 1 or 2

Egg suppers, for one or two people, are even easier and quicker than frittatas. They are a Sunday evening favorite in my family. Use the same ingredients as you would for a frittata, including the ones on pages 203 to 204, only instead of beating the eggs, make shallow depressions in the ingredients in the pan and break an egg into each depression. Then add the remaining ingredients, cover the skillet, and cook over very low heat until the eggs are done to your taste.

    2 teaspoons unsalted butter
    1 10-ounce carton frozen spinach, defrosted
    salt
    freshly ground pepper
    2 eggs
    Worcestershire sauce
    4 tablespoons grated cheddar

Melt the butter in an 8-inch nonstick skillet over moderate heat. With your hands, squeeze the liquid out of the spinach leaves, add the leaves to the pan, and stir until well heated. Season with salt and pepper to taste. Spread out the spinach and make 2 depressions in it. Break an egg into each depression, and sprinkle drops of Worcestershire sauce and 2 tablespoons of grated cheddar over each yolk. Cover the pan, lower the heat, and cook slowly until the eggs are done to your taste.

Asparagus and Ham Egg Supper

Use the same ingredients as in Asparagus and Ham Frittata (page 203) and cook the asparagus and ham as directed. Create 2 or 3 open spaces among the asparagus slices and break an egg into each one. Sprinkle with salt and pepper to taste and add a few drops of Worcestershire sauce to each egg yolk, if you like. Dust with grated Gruyère, or not. Cover the pan, lower the heat, and cook slowly until the eggs are done to your taste.

BROILED SALMON FILLET

❖

Serves 3 or 4

1 to 1¼ pounds salmon fillet
1 tablespoon soy sauce
1 tablespoon mirin or sherry
1 tablespoon Dijon mustard
1 large clove garlic, peeled and very thinly sliced
very thinly sliced lemon rounds, cut into quarters,
    or 2 Preserved Lemon quarters (page 190),
    rinsed and cut into slivers
Green Sauce (page 192, optional)

Preheat the broiler.

Combine the soy sauce, mirin and mustard and brush over the top of the salmon. Distribute the sliced garlic and lemon over the top of the fillet. Place a cast-iron skillet large enough to hold the salmon over high heat. When the skillet is very hot, place the salmon in it, skin side down, and cook for about 3 minutes, or until the bottom of the salmon is partially cooked. Place the pan under the broiler and broil for 3 to 5 minutes, depending on the thickness of the fillet and how well done you want it to be. The salmon will con-

tinue to cook for a few minutes once it's out of the broiler. Serve with lemon
wedges and green sauce, if desired.

POACHED SALMON

❖

Serves 4 or 5

I first made this recipe for my mother, who thought it was delicious and del-
icate. It's perfect for company, and so easy to prepare! Chicken broth makes
a quick and tasty poaching medium for salmon and other fish, and it's even
better with a little wine added. Be sure to reserve the poaching liquid for Fish
and Corn Chowder (page 199) or for the risotto on page 215.

> chicken broth
> dry white wine (optional)
> salt
> 1¼ to 1½ pounds salmon fillet
> thinly sliced lemon, or finely minced rind of Preserved
>   Lemon (page 190) and small capers (optional)
> Green Sauce (page 192) or Yogurt with Garlic and Cucumber
>   (page 194)

Place the salmon in a skillet or other flameproof vessel just large enough to
hold it and add water to cover. Remove the salmon and measure the water to
see how much poaching liquid you will need—probably between 4 and 6
cups. Add the requisite amount of chicken broth plus an additional cup or
half-cup of dry white wine or water and salt to taste to the skillet and bring
it to a boil. Return the salmon to the skillet and bring to a simmer over high
heat. Lower the heat, cover the skillet, and simmer the fish gently until it is
barely opaque when a sharp knife is inserted into the thickest part of the fillet, about 10 minutes for a fillet that is 1 inch thick.

Remove the salmon with one or two large slotted spatulas and place on a platter or individual plates. Decorate with lemon and capers, if you wish. Serve hot or cold with green sauce or with the yogurt and cucumbers. If serving cold, cover the fish as it cools to prevent the top from drying out.

BEAN AND TUNA SALAD VINAIGRETTE

❖

Serves 3 as lunch dish, 4 as a first course

Most of us have at least one or two cans of tuna on hand. It's one of the most healthful convenience foods we have—a great source of omega-3 fatty acids and also good-quality protein—and there is so much you can do with it. Follow your own taste in selecting tuna—some people like it packed in olive oil, others prefer the kind that's water-packed.

In Mediterranean countries, any of the salads that follow might be spooned into ripe, hollowed-out tomatoes and served either as a first course or as one of several luncheon dishes, at room temperature. If you are going to use either of the bean and tuna salads as a filling for tomatoes, omit the cherry tomatoes and substitute ¼ cup chopped pitted black olives.

1 15-ounce can cannellini or chickpeas
½ cup diced or coarsely chopped celery
½ cup chopped red onion
generous ½ cup halved cherry or grape tomatoes
1 tablespoon tiny capers
1 6-ounce can tuna fish in olive oil or water
   (preferably imported), drained
2 or 3 tablespoons chopped flat parsley
1 tablespoon fresh lemon juice
1 tablespoon balsamic vinegar
2 tablespoons extra-virgin olive oil

salt
freshly ground pepper

Drain the beans in a sieve, rinse briefly under cold running water, then drain again. Place the beans in a bowl and add the celery, onion, tomatoes, capers, tuna, and parsley. Toss lightly. Combine the lemon juice, vinegar, oil, and salt and pepper to taste, and pour over the beans and tuna. Mix just until combined; try not to tear the tuna into fine shreds.

Serve cold or at room temperature.

Cannellini and Tuna Salad with Basil Vinaigrette

Prepare the bean and tuna mixture using cannellini beans. To make the dressing, place ½ cup packed basil leaves and one small to medium peeled garlic clove in a blender or food processor and chop fine. Add the lemon juice, vinegar, oil, and salt and pepper to taste and blend until the mixture is pureed. If the dressing is too thick, add one or two tablespoons of water and blend again. Pour over the bean mixture and combine lightly.

TUNA SALAD WITH PRESERVED LEMON

❖

Serves 2

1 6-ounce can tuna fish packed in oil or water
   (preferably imported), drained
⅓ cup chopped red or Vidalia onion
2 tablespoons chopped red bell pepper
2 teaspoons tiny capers
1 quarter Preserved Lemon (page 190), rinsed and minced
2 tablespoons chopped fresh coriander
2 to 3 teaspoons lemon juice

2 tablespoons extra-virgin olive oil

salt

freshly ground pepper

Place the tuna in a bowl and add the onion, red pepper, capers, preserved lemon, and coriander. Toss lightly. Combine the lemon juice, oil, and salt and pepper to taste and pour over the tuna. Mix just until combined. Serve on a bed of greens or toss with salad greens.

CORNISH HENS WITH WHEATBERRY STUFFING

❖

Serves 2

3 tablespoons Honey Mustard–Balsamic Vinegar Glaze
   (page 197)

2 Cornish hens, about 1 pound each

1 cup Wheatberries with Fruit and Honey-Orange Dressing
   (page 212)

2 teaspoons chopped fresh tarragon or ½ teaspoon dried
   tarragon

olive oil

juice of ½ orange

salt

freshly ground pepper

Preheat the oven to 425° F.

Rub the glaze all over the hens, inside and out, reserving any that remains. Combine the wheatberry salad with the tarragon and stuff the hens loosely with the mixture. Place the hens on a rack in a shallow, flame-proof baking pan (I use a cast-iron skillet, which is easy to deglaze), brush with oil, and roast until they are deep golden brown and the thigh bones move easily in their sockets, about 40 minutes. Brush the birds with the reserved glaze and with oil twice during roasting.

Transfer the birds to a platter or individual plates and remove the rack from the pan. Place the pan over medium heat and add the orange juice and any remaining glaze, scraping up all the browned bits at the bottom of the pan with a spatula. Reduce the sauce until about ¼ cup remains, taste for seasoning, and spoon over the birds. Serve at once.

CHICKEN BREASTS WITH SQUASH, TOMATOES, AND PRESERVED LEMON

❖

Serves 4

This is simply a very quick summer vegetable stew cooked with chicken breasts. Of course, you can substitute an equal amount of boneless turkey breast or freshly made, nitrate-free chicken sausages.

2 small yellow squash (about 12 ounces)
2 small zucchini (about 12 ounces)
2 tablespoons olive oil
2 10- to 12-ounce boneless, skinless whole chicken breasts,
    cut in half
1 cup finely chopped shallots or onions
1 or 2 large cloves garlic, peeled and minced
2 cups canned tomatoes (preferably organic), with juices
1 tablespoon chopped fresh ginger
large pinch cayenne or hot or mild paprika
salt
freshly ground pepper
2 or 3 quarters Preserved Lemon (page 190), rinsed and
    chopped
¼ cup chopped fresh mint
¼ cup chopped fresh coriander

Trim the squash and zucchini and cut into ¾-inch diagonal slices. If the squash are very thick, cut them in half lengthwise and then into diagonal slices. Set aside. Heat 1 tablespoon of oil in a large heavy skillet over moderate heat, add the chicken, and brown lightly on both sides. Transfer to a plate and reserve. Add the remaining tablespoon of oil to the skillet, add the shallots and garlic, and brown lightly. Add the remaining ingredients except the chicken and stir, scraping up all the browned bits on the bottom of the pan. Cover the pan and cook for about 5 minutes. Taste for seasoning. Return the chicken breasts to the pan, spoon some of the sauce over them, and cook, covered, over moderately low heat for 10 minutes, or until the chicken is just cooked; do not overcook. The squash should still have some crunch. Turn the breasts in the sauce after 5 minutes. Taste for seasoning and serve over whole wheat couscous or brown rice.

Monkfish with Squash, Tomatoes, and Preserved Lemon

Substitute 1¼ to 1½ pounds of monkfish for the chicken, but do not add it until the sauce is made. Cut the fish into ⅝-inch thick medallions. After the squash and tomatoes have cooked for 10 minutes, add the monkfish and bury it in the sauce. Cook 5 minutes longer, or until the fish is just cooked and the squash is still firm to the bite.

WHEATBERRIES WITH FRUIT AND HONEY-ORANGE DRESSING

❖

Makes 3½ to 4 cups

This recipe introduced me to wheatberries. It has already become a staple in our house. It's easy to make and my husband loves it. I like this pilaf best made with soft wheatberries, which cook up to a beautiful pale color and a tender but crunchy texture in about 30 minutes after soaking. The dish is delicious served by itself, but I also love it for breakfast topped with some *honey-sweetened low-fat yogurt, as an accompaniment to meats and poultry, as part of a buffet, or used as a stuffing for Cornish hens (page 210). It's also an inspired filling for Oma's Easter Grain Pie on page 236.*

You'll need a sharp paring knife to cut up the fruit.

1 cup summer (soft) white wheatberries, spelt, or farro
salt
1 orange
½ cup dried cranberries, coarsely chopped
½ cup dried (unsulfured) apricots, cut into thin slivers
6 tablespoons pine nuts
4 teaspoons honey

You can soak the wheatberries overnight in water to cover by about an inch or you can place them in a heavy medium saucepan, add water to cover by at least an inch, and bring to a boil. Cover the pan, turn off the heat, and let the berries sit for two hours. Drain the soaked berries, return to the pan, and cover with at least an inch of fresh water. Bring to a boil over high heat, lower the heat, and cook the berries, covered, at a gentle boil for about 30 minutes, or until the grain is cooked but still crunchy. Add salt to taste 10 minutes or more before the grain is done. Drain the wheatberries and transfer to a bowl. You will have a generous 2½ cups.

Remove the zest from the orange in long strips, using a vegetable peeler. Cut 8 or 9 strips of it into very thin slivers, then cut the slivers into tiny dice. Add to the wheatberries with the cranberries, apricots, and pine nuts. Squeeze the orange into a small bowl. In another bowl, whisk 4 tablespoons of the juice into the honey and add to the pilaf. Mix well and taste for salt, which, added in very small amounts, brings out the flavor of the fruit.

Serve warm, at room temperature, or cold. If using for stuffing, let the grain come to room temperature before spooning it into the bird. Store, well covered, in the refrigerator for up to three days, or in the freezer for one month.

PUFFED CORNMEAL PANCAKE
WITH CRANBERRIES

❖

Makes 1 10-inch pancake

*E*ach of these pancakes is a delicious weekend breakfast treat. If you like,
you can sprinkle the baked cranberry pancake with confectioner's sugar
and serve it as a dessert. Use the corn pancake as a side dish or as a very light
main course.

¼ cup stone-ground cornmeal
¼ cup all-purpose flour
1 teaspoon baking powder
½ teaspoon salt
2 large eggs, separated
1 egg white
½ cup milk
½ cup dried cranberries
1 tablespoon safflower or canola oil or butter
1 tablespoon sugar
maple syrup or honey

Preheat the oven to 400° F. Place a 10-inch skillet (I use seasoned cast-iron)
in the oven to preheat.

Combine the cornmeal, flour, baking powder, and salt on a sheet of wax
paper and set aside. In a mixing bowl, with an electric mixer, beat the yolks
at high speed until thickened, then beat in the milk. Stir in the dry ingredients and the cranberries.

Add the oil to the preheated skillet and return to the oven. With clean
beaters, beat the egg whites at high speed until they are foamy, gradually add
the sugar, and beat until soft peaks form. Stir one quarter of the whites into
the batter, then fold in the rest. Pour the batter into the skillet and bake the

pancake for 15 minutes, or until puffed and golden. Serve from pan at once with syrup or honey.

Puffed Cornmeal Pancake with Fresh Corn and Cheddar

Omit the cranberries. Instead, add the kernels from 1 ear of corn (⅔ to ¾ cup, or use frozen corn); ½ jalapeño pepper, stemmed, cored, and minced; 2 ounces cheddar cheese, grated (about ½ cup); and a pinch of cayenne. Proceed as directed. Serve at once.

BARLEY RISOTTO WITH SHRIMP AND EDAMAME

❖

Serves 4

A rich stock makes all the difference in this recipe. I always freeze the poaching liquid from salmon (page 207) or other poached fish dishes, but if you don't have any on hand, use chicken stock or canned chicken broth and augment it with the shrimp shells. Barley, with its delicious flavor and interesting texture, is an excellent substitute for arborio rice in this risotto, and it requires almost no attention after it's begun to cook.

1 pound large shrimp
2 cups chicken broth or fish stock
1 or 2 sprigs fresh dill or parsley (optional)
1 to 2 tablespoons unsalted butter
1 or 2 shallots, minced
1 clove garlic, minced
1 cup pearled barley, rinsed and drained
salt
freshly ground pepper
1½ cups frozen shelled edamame

Shell the shrimp and reserve them, covered, in the refrigerator. Place the shrimp shells, chicken broth, dill, if using, and 2 cups of water in a medium saucepan and bring to a boil over moderately high heat. Reduce the heat and cook the broth, covered, at a rapid simmer for about 20 minutes, or until the shells have imparted their flavor and the broth is somewhat reduced. Strain the broth; you should have about 3½ cups. Reserve.

In a large skillet or nonstick wok, melt 1 tablespoon of the butter over moderate heat, add the shallot and garlic, and sauté until the shallot is translucent, about 3 minutes. Add the barley, 3 cups of the reserved broth, and salt and pepper to taste, and bring to a boil. Cover the pan, reduce the heat to low, and simmer the barley for about 20 minutes, or until it is almost tender. (Some barley takes up to 40 minutes to cook, so read the package instructions.) Stir in the edamame and shelled shrimp and cook, covered, for 6 to 8 minutes, or just until the shrimp are pink. Fold in the remaining tablespoon (or less) of butter and taste for seasoning. Serve hot.

Barley Risotto with Wild Mushrooms and Edamame

Omit the shrimp and use instead 6 to 8 ounces shiitake mushrooms, stemmed and cut into ½-inch pieces, or oyster mushrooms, ends trimmed and cut into ½-inch cubes. In a skillet or wok, sauté the mushrooms in 1 tablespoon of the butter for 3 to 5 minutes, remove from the skillet and reserve. Proceed with the recipe, using 3 cups of chicken or vegetable stock. After the edamame are almost cooked, add the mushrooms and reheat. Fold in ¼ cup of grated Parmesan just before serving.

BROWN RICE SALAD WITH GREEN VEGETABLES

❖

Serves 2

*P*reserved lemon gives this salad a special zing. Use leftover steamed broccoli rape or set aside some of the Broccoli Rape with Garlic and Bell Pepper (page 224), Stir-Fried Green Vegetables and Mushrooms (page 228), or
Edamame Salad (page 230). Steamed broccoli, string beans, roasted vegetables, and summer squash are all fine. This salad doesn't need much dressing
since most of the vegetables will already have absorbed some of the oil they
were cooked in.

1 cup or more cooked broccoli or other cooked green
     vegetables, cut into ½-inch pieces, if necessary
1 cup or more cooked brown rice
5 or 6 grape or cherry tomatoes, halved
1 small garlic clove, minced
chopped red onion to taste
1 quarter Preserved Lemon (page 190), rinsed and minced,
     or mild vinegar to taste
1 tablespoon extra-virgin olive oil

Combine all the ingredients in a bowl and serve at once. In this salad, the
sum vastly exceeds the parts in flavor.

CURRIED BROWN RICE SALAD

❖

Serves 4 to 6 as a first course or side dish

Another good reason for cooking more brown rice than you can eat at one meal.

Dressing

1 tablespoon good-quality mayonnaise (I use Hellmann's
    Real Mayonnaise)
¼ cup low-fat or nonfat plain yogurt
1 tablespoon rice wine vinegar or other mild vinegar
salt
freshly ground pepper
½ teaspoon curry powder

Salad

1 cup cold cooked brown rice
handful of chopped fresh dill and/or parsley
⅓ cup chopped red onion
⅓ cup chopped celery
⅓ cup chopped red or green bell pepper
1 4- or 5-ounce apple, quartered, cored, and cut
    into ⅜-inch dice
3 tablespoons currants or chopped dried cranberries
3 tablespoons toasted sunflower seeds

For the dressing, combine all the ingredients and mix well.

Place the rice in a mixing bowl, breaking up any clumps with a fork or your hands. Add the remaining salad ingredients and toss lightly. Add the dressing as soon as the apple is mixed into the salad and stir gently. Cover well and allow the flavors to blend for at least 30 minutes and up to 1 day. Serve cold or at room temperature.

BROCCOLI AND BROWN RICE CASSEROLE

❖

Serves 4 to 6

This is a healthy dish, easy to assemble, and very tasty.

2 cups cooked brown rice
¾ cup Marinara Sauce (page 193) or good-quality canned
    tomato sauce
1 cup part-skim ricotta
2 tablespoons chopped fresh basil or parsley
2½ to 3 cups chopped cooked broccoli (1 bunch,
    including peeled stems)
salt
freshly ground pepper
generous ½ cup grated cheddar cheese
¼ cup grated Parmesan cheese

Preheat the oven to 350° F. Oil a 2-quart casserole.

Combine the rice and marinara sauce and spread in the bottom of the casserole. Combine the ricotta and basil and spread over the rice. Season the broccoli with salt and pepper to taste and distribute evenly over the ricotta. Sprinkle the top with the cheddar and Parmesan and bake for 20 to 30 minutes, or until very hot.

WHOLE-WHEAT COUSCOUS

❖

Serves 5 or 6

*I*nstant couscous is widely available now in supermarkets, very often packaged with seasonings and instructions for preparing the grain. This recipe
calls for whole-wheat semolina couscous, which you can buy at Middle
Eastern and health-food stores (see the Resources section) and which tastes
delicious, especially if you use stock or broth for the liquid.

> 2 tablespoons olive oil
> 1 cup whole-wheat couscous
> 2 cups boiling water, chicken stock, or canned chicken broth
> pinch saffron (optional)
> salt

Heat the olive oil in a heavy saucepan over a medium flame, add the couscous, and stir for a minute or two, until the oil is absorbed. Add the boiling
liquid, saffron, if using, and salt to taste. Stir the couscous, cover the pot, and
simmer over low heat for 5 to 10 minutes, or until all the liquid is absorbed.
Fluff up the grain with a fork. Serve hot or at room temperature.

Whole-Wheat Couscous with Roasted Vegetables

Fold in 2 cups roasted vegetables, such as Roasted Brussels Sprouts with Carrots and Shallots (page 225), cut into bite-size pieces if necessary. Cover the
pan so that the vegetables can absorb heat from the grain. Serve warm or at
room temperature.

Black Bean Salad with Tomato, Avocado, and Lime Dressing

❖

Serves 3 or 4

This is a good, quick recipe that I make whenever I find ripe avocados at the market. Eat the salad the same day you make it—before the avocado turns color.

1 15-ounce can black beans
½ cup diced red onion
½ cup diced green or red bell pepper
½ jalapeño pepper, cored, seeded, and minced (optional)
½ cup quartered grape or cherry tomatoes
½ Hass avocado, cut into dice
2 tablespoons chopped fresh coriander

Dressing

2 tablespoons fresh lime juice
1 teaspoon sherry vinegar
1½ tablespoons extra-virgin olive oil
½ teaspoon ground cumin
Salt
Freshly ground black pepper

Drain the beans, rinse them very briefly under cold running water, and drain again. Transfer them to a bowl, add onion, bell pepper, jalapeño pepper (if using), tomato, avocado, and coriander, and toss lightly.

Combine all the dressing ingredients in a small bowl and whisk until well mixed. Add the dressing to the beans mixture and stir gently. Cover the salad with wax paper or plastic wrap and allow the flavors to blend for 1 or 2 hours at room temperature or in refrigerator. Bring the salad back to room temperature before serving.

FARMSTAND TOMATO SALAD

❖

Serves 4 or 5

This seasonal first course—closer to a soup than a salad—should be made during the one month a year when locally grown, freshly picked, heirloom tomatoes are out on the farmstands. But during that month, you can eat it every day! Instead of serving the salad over bread, you can also use it as a pasta sauce.

1¼ to 1½ pounds red and yellow heirloom tomatoes
1 large garlic clove, peeled and chopped
½ red onion, peeled, halved, thinly sliced, and separated
    into rings
8 to 10 fresh basil leaves
salt
freshly ground black pepper
3 tablespoons fruity extra-virgin olive oil
2 tablespoons balsamic vinegar
4 or 5 thin slices crusty whole-grain bread

Core the tomatoes, cut them in half horizontally, and cut each half into ½-inch wedges. Put the tomatoes into a bowl and add the garlic and onion. Wash the basil leaves, then stack them up and cut them into lengthwise strips. Add to the bowl. Combine salt and pepper to taste with the olive oil and vinegar, pour over the tomatoes, and toss gently. Let the salad stand for about 15 minutes until the tomatoes release their juices.

Tear the bread into bite-size pieces and distribute among 4 or 5 shallow soup plates. Ladle the tomato salad over the bread, allow the juices to soak into the bread for 10 to 15 minutes, and serve.

CARROT SALAD

❖

Serves 4

We love raw carrots in my family; they are so healthful and fresh-tasting. This salad is a welcome change from the usual carrot sticks, and the raspberry vinegar adds a bright note to the flavor. If you have a fine shredder attachment for your processor, use it for the carrots—they'll taste even sweeter and juicier.

8 ounces carrots, trimmed, peeled, and grated (preferably in
   a food processor to get the longest slivers)
2 tablespoons snipped dill
2 scallions, trimmed and thinly sliced (optional)
1½ tablespoons extra-virgin olive oil
1 tablespoon raspberry vinegar
½ teaspoon ground cumin
pinch sugar
salt

Combine the carrots, dill, and scallions, if using, in a bowl. Whisk together the oil, vinegar, cumin, sugar, and salt to taste. Mix with the carrots. Serve at room temperature or cold.

BROCCOLI RABE WITH GARLIC
AND BELL PEPPER

❖

Serves 4

B roccoli rabe, a deep-green, leafy member of the broccoli (crucifer) family, cooks very quickly—5 or 6 minutes in all. It has a more pronounced flavor than broccoli (because most of the flavor has been bred out of broccoli by now); however, if you cook the green in a lot of water it will have a milder flavor. Since I prefer that extra bite, I cook it in only a half inch of water. I usually cook extra broccoli rabe without garlic and bell peppers as a planned leftover to use in salads, with grains, or simply drizzled with olive oil. The recipe below is delicious on its own and also makes a terrific sauce for pasta such as penne rigate or rigatoni, with freshly grated Parmesan to complete the dish.

> 1 bunch broccoli rabe (1 to 1½ pounds)
> salt
> 2 tablespoons olive oil
> 1 or 2 large garlic cloves, peeled and minced
> red pepper flakes (optional)
> ½ red bell pepper, stemmed, seeded, and diced

Bring either 2 or 3 quarts (for a milder flavor) or ½ inch (for a stronger flavor) of water to boil in a large covered saucepan. Cut off and discard the broccoli rabe stem bottoms and rinse the vegetable under running water. Cut the stems into 1-inch lengths, then cut the leaf and bud portion into 2- or 3-inch lengths. When the water comes to a boil, add salt to taste, add the broccoli stems, and cook, covered, for 2 to 3 minutes, or until half tender. Add the broccoli tops, stir down in the pan until they have wilted a little, cover, and cook for another 2 to 4 minutes, or until the vegetable is just cooked. Drain in a colander, and place under cold running water briefly to set the color and stop the cooking. Drain again and transfer to a serving dish.

In a small skillet, heat the oil over medium heat. Add the garlic and red pepper flakes, if using, and fry briefly until the garlic is cooked to your taste, depending on how raw a flavor you like—the strong taste of the broccoli rape won't be overwhelmed by a strong flavor of garlic. Add the bell pepper and stir for a minute or two in the hot oil until the pepper has softened a little. Scrape the mixture out on top of the broccoli rabe and serve at once or at room temperature.

ROASTED BRUSSELS SPROUTS WITH CARROTS AND SHALLOTS

❖

Serves 4

Until my stepmother, Lisa, showed me how to roast Brussels sprouts, I always thought of them as watery, mushy minicabbages with no flavor at all. Now all that's changed, and I serve them often, especially in the fall when I buy them on the stem at farmstands.

    16 to 20 Brussels sprouts
    20 baby carrots
    4 large shallots, peeled and halved
    salt
    olive oil

Preheat the oven to 450° F.

Trim the bottoms of the sprouts, pull off and discard any wilted or yellow leaves. Place the sprouts and carrots and shallots, if using, on a cookie sheet, jelly roll pan, or heavy skillet, sprinkle with salt, and drizzle with 1 or 2 teaspoons of olive oil. Rub the oil and salt into the vegetables and spread them out in the pan; don't overcrowd or they'll steam instead of roasting. Roast for 15 to 20 minutes, turning once, or until the sprouts are nicely browned on two sides, but still quite crunchy. Serve hot, warm, or at room temperature.

This is also good used for Whole-Wheat Couscous with Roasted Vegetables (page 220).

ROASTED SLICED BRUSSELS SPROUTS WITH GARLIC AND ONION

❖

Serves 4

My family loves this recipe.

> 1 pint (about 10 ounces) Brussels sprouts
> 1 medium onion, peeled and sliced
> 1 garlic clove, peeled and minced
> salt
> olive oil

Preheat the oven to 450° F.

Remove any wilted or yellowed leaves from the Brussels sprouts and trim the stems close to the heads. Cut each head vertically into thin slices and put them on a baking sheet or heavy skillet. Break the onion slices apart into rings and add to the sprouts along with the garlic and a light sprinkling of salt. Spray generously or drizzle with olive oil, toss the vegetables to coat them lightly with oil, and spread out evenly on the baking sheet or skillet. Bake for about 15 minutes, or until the vegetables are lightly browned and tender, stirring once or twice as they roast. I usually serve this recipe with brown rice or couscous.

LENTILS WITH FRIED ONIONS

❖

Serves 6 to 8

When you add water to the pan in which you've caramelized the onions, you'll have a very mild, but still flavorful, onion soup in which to cook the lentils. They are a classic accompaniment to brown rice or any whole grain.

2 tablespoons olive oil
1 pound onions, peeled, quartered and sliced
1 cup brown or green lentils
salt

Pour the oil into a heavy skillet (I use a 10-inch cast-iron) or saucepan and place over moderate heat. Add the onions and cook, stirring often, until they are tender, starting to become crisp, and have turned a rich brown color. This can take as long as 20 minutes. Remove half the onions to a dish and reserve. Add the lentils, salt to taste, and water to barely cover the lentils. Bring to a boil, stirring up the caramelized bits of onion at the bottom of the skillet. Lower the heat, and simmer the lentils and onions for about 25 minutes, covered, or until the lentils are cooked but still firm to the bite. Check a few times to see that there is enough water; add it sparingly, if necessary. If there is too much liquid, remove the cover and boil the lentils to evaporate excess water. Stir in the reserved onions and taste for seasoning. Serve hot or at room temperature.

STIR-FRIED GREEN VEGETABLES AND MUSHROOMS

❖

Serves 5 or 6

This recipe takes less than 10 minutes to prepare and it always looks beautiful, especially with the browned sesame seeds, which also add a nutty crunch to the dish. Good green-vegetable-and-mushroom combinations are: asparagus with oyster mushrooms, green beans or sugar snaps (or both) with white mushrooms, snow peas with shiitakes. Use any leftovers in a brown rice salad (page 217) or in a frittata (pages 203–204).

  1 tablespoon sesame seeds
  1 tablespoon safflower oil
  1-inch piece ginger, peeled and cut into slivers
  1 pound asparagus, green beans, snow peas, or sugar snap
     peas, trimmed and cut into 1-inch diagonal slices
  6 to 8 ounces mushrooms (white, oyster, shiitake, cremini,
     etc.), trimmed and sliced or cut into bite-size pieces
  4 scallions, trimmed and sliced diagonally
  1 tablespoon mirin or sherry
  1 tablespoon soy sauce
  salt
  freshly ground pepper

In a heavy skillet or dry wok, preferably nonstick, toast the sesame seeds over moderately high heat until lightly browned, shaking the pan and stirring the seeds—they burn very fast. Scrape the seeds into a bowl. Add 1½ teaspoons of oil to the pan; add the ginger and stir-fry for about 30 seconds; then add the green vegetable and stir-fry for 2 to 3 minutes, or until cooked but still very crunchy. Transfer the mixture to the bowl with the sesame seeds. Add remaining 1½ teaspoons of oil to pan; add the mushrooms and stir-fry for 1 or 2 minutes; add the scallions and stir; return vegetables and sesame seeds to pan and toss until hot. Add mirin, soy sauce, and salt and pepper to taste, and cook a few seconds longer. Serve at once or at room temperature.

Stir-Fried Green Vegetables and Mushrooms with Tofu

Cut a 12-ounce cake of extra-firm tofu into ½-inch cubes. Add to the mushrooms with the vegetables and sesame seeds and increase the soy sauce and mirin to 2 tablespoons each. Serve with brown rice.

SOYFUL SUCCOTASH

❖

Serves 4

This is a luxurious recipe, meant either for special occasions or for those times when the rest of the meal is somewhat austere. Of course, you can make it with frozen corn, but fresh off the cob is best by far.

3 ears corn
2 cups frozen shelled edamame
1 cup half-and-half
pinch salt
2 teaspoons unsalted butter
2 tablespoons grated Parmesan or Jack cheese (optional)

Shuck the corn and cut the kernels off the cobs with a sharp paring knife; you should have about 2 cups of kernels. Put the kernels into a heavy medium saucepan with the edamame, half-and-half, and salt and bring to a boil. Cook, uncovered, at a medium boil for 5 or 6 minutes, or until the cream is reduced by at least half. Fold in the butter and the cheese, if using. Taste for seasoning and serve at once.

SUPERQUICK SOYFUL SUCCOTASH

❖

Serves 4

This healthy soy succotash is a dish you can make all year round. It is simple and fresh-tasting. Edamame and corn are such a natural pairing that
you will find yourself serving it often. You can also use it in the Edamame
Salad that follows.

  2 cups frozen corn kernels
  2 cups frozen shelled edamame
  salt
  2 teaspoons unsalted butter

Place the corn and edamame in a medium saucepan, add ¾ to 1 cup of water
and salt to taste and bring to a boil. Cook uncovered for about 3 to 4 minutes, drain, and place in a bowl. Fold in the butter and serve at once.

EDAMAME SALAD

❖

Serves 4

Mild rice wine vinegar is a good complement to the subtle flavor of the
soybeans.

  2 cups (10 ounces) frozen shelled edamame
  salt
  ⅓ cup finely chopped sweet or red onion
  ¼ cup chopped fresh dill

1 tablespoon rice wine vinegar
1½ tablespoons extra-virgin olive oil
freshly ground white pepper

In a small saucepan, bring the edamame, about ½ cup of water, and salt to taste to a boil over high heat. Reduce the flame, cover the pan, and cook for 2 or 3 minutes, or until just tender. Drain the beans, and put them into a bowl of cold water to stop the cooking and set the color. When they are cool, drain well and transfer to a bowl. Add the onion and dill. Shake the vinegar, oil, pepper, and salt, if needed, in a small jar, add to the edamame, and mix well. Serve at room temperature.

STEAMED EDAMAME IN THE SHELL

❖

This is my family's favorite snack, the one I serve to everyone who passes through the house. The cooked pods are a beautiful rich green, and it's fun to slit them open and eat those delicious beans right out of the shell!

8 to 16 ounces frozen edamame in the pod
salt

Place the beans in a medium saucepan, add 1 to 1½ cups of water and salt to taste (the beans need quite a bit of salt), and bring to a boil over high heat. Cover and simmer the beans for 3 to 5 minutes, or until they are just cooked—they become mushy fast. Remove one of the pods from the pot, chill it in cold water, and taste the beans. If they are just tender, the beans are done. Drain the pods and place in a bowl of cold water to stop the cooking and set the color. Drain again and serve. The beans will keep for 1 or 2 days, well covered, in the refrigerator. (We never have any left over.)

MIM'S MELTAWAYS

❖

Makes 40 to 45 cookies

Judy developed these cookies for me because I love nuts and have a soft spot for cookies. The cookies freeze well, but they might need an extra dusting of confectioner's sugar before serving.

¾ cup ground unblanched hazelnuts or blanched almonds
¼ cup whole-wheat flour
½ cup all-purpose flour
4 ounces (1 stick) unsalted butter, at room temperature
½ cup confectioner's sugar, plus more for sifting
grated zest of 1 orange
1 teaspoon vanilla extract

Combine the hazelnuts and whole wheat and white flours and set aside. In a mixing bowl with an electric mixer, beat the butter until it is light. Add the confectioner's sugar and orange zest and beat until fluffy. Beat in the vanilla. Add the dry ingredients and mix very well, scraping down the sides of the bowl as necessary. Cover with wax paper, and refrigerate for about 30 minutes, or until firm enough to handle.

Preheat the oven to 350° F. Grease cookie sheets or line with parchment paper (the paper is easier to handle).

Shape the dough into balls ¾-inch to 1 inch in diameter and place 1½ inches apart on the cookie sheets. Bake in the middle of the oven for about 15 minutes, or until golden around the edges, rotating the pans halfway through baking. Cool the cookies for 2 to 3 minutes on the pans, then carefully slide them off onto a sheet of wax paper placed on a piece of clean newspaper, or simply slide the parchment paper off the cookie sheet onto the newspaper. Sift confectioner's sugar over the cookies while they are still warm. The cookies are fragile while hot, so don't handle until they are cool.

WALNUT ZUCCHINI BREAD

❖

Makes 1 8-inch loaf

The bread freezes very well, so you might want to make a couple while you're up and about. I serve this cakelike bread as a dessert—it's moist and delicious and filled with good things.

¾ cup whole-wheat flour
¾ cup unbleached flour
1 teaspoon baking soda
½ teaspoon baking powder
pinch salt
1 teaspoon cinnamon
2 eggs
¾ cup sugar
⅓ cup safflower or canola oil
¼ cup fresh orange juice
2 tablespoons plain low-fat or nonfat yogurt
1 teaspoon vanilla extract
grated zest of 1 orange
grated zest of 1 lemon
1 cup grated zucchini
1 cup chopped walnuts, pecans, or hazelnuts

Preheat the oven to 350° F. Butter and sugar an 8-inch loaf pan.

Sift the flours, baking soda, baking powder, salt, and cinnamon onto a piece of wax paper. In a large mixing bowl with an electric mixer (hand-held, if you like; this bread doesn't require heavy beating), beat the eggs and sugar until well mixed and slightly thickened. Beat in the oil, juice, yogurt, vanilla, and grated zests. Add the dry ingredients, zucchini, and nuts and beat by hand until well mixed. Pour the batter into the prepared pan and bake for 50 minutes, or until deep golden brown. Cool on a rack.

Apple Hazelnut Bread

Substitute apple juice for the orange juice. Instead of zucchini, just before adding it, core a medium apple (no need to peel it) and chop it in a food processor or by hand. Measure 1 cup and add immediately to the batter along with 1 cup of chopped hazelnuts.

CARROT MUFFINS

❖

Makes 12 muffins

This recipe is a variation on Walnut Zucchini Bread. The muffins freeze very well.

¾ cup whole-wheat flour
1 cup unbleached flour
1 teaspoon baking soda
½ teaspoon baking powder
pinch salt
1 teaspoon cinnamon
2 eggs
¾ cup sugar
⅓ cup safflower or canola oil
¼ cup fresh orange juice
¼ cup plain nonfat yogurt
1 teaspoon vanilla extract
grated zest of ½ orange
1 cup, packed, grated raw carrot
½ cup raisins
1 cup chopped walnuts, pecans, or hazelnuts

Preheat the oven to 350° F. Butter 12 muffin tins.

Sift the flours, baking soda, baking powder, salt, and cinnamon onto a piece of wax paper. In a large mixing bowl with an electric mixer (hand-held, if you like; this batter doesn't require heavy beating), beat the eggs and sugar until well mixed and slightly thickened. Beat in the oil, juice, yogurt, vanilla, and grated zest. Add the dry ingredients, carrot, raisins, and nuts and beat by hand until well mixed. Pour the batter into the prepared tins and bake for 20 to 25 minutes, or until deep golden brown. Cool on a rack.

FRUIT CRISP

❖

Serves 8

½ cup old-fashioned rolled oats
1 cup fresh whole-wheat bread crumbs
½ cup, packed, dark brown sugar
½ cup chopped nuts
5 tablespoons unsalted butter
juice of 1 lemon
2 pounds pears or apples or (preferably) both
½ cup dried cranberries
½ teaspoon cinnamon
½ teaspoon allspice
¼ teaspoon freshly grated nutmeg
¼ cup apple juice

Preheat the oven to 350° F. Butter a shallow baking dish or a 9-inch pie plate.

In a mixing bowl, combine the oatmeal, bread crumbs, sugar, and nuts and mix well. Melt the butter in a large skillet or wok, add the oatmeal mixture and mix well. Reserve. Pour the lemon juice into the mixing bowl. Peel, quarter, core, and slice the pears and/or apples and add them to the bowl, tossing to coat the slices with lemon juice. Add the spices and toss again. Arrange the fruit in the baking dish, sprinkle the layers with the cranberries, and pour the lemon juice and apple juice over the fruit. Spread the oat mixture evenly over the fruit and bake for about 40 minutes, or until the fruit is soft. Serve warm or at room temperature, with ice cream, if you like.

OMA'S EASTER GRAIN PIE

❖

Makes 1 9-inch pie, serving 8 to 10

I *often freeze leftover whole-grain bread to make into bread crumbs for this recipe and for the Fruit Crisp on the previous page. Oma was the mother of Judy's good friend Rosemarie, who makes this pie every Easter.*

1 tablespoon unsalted butter, softened
¼ cup coarse whole-grain bread crumbs
4 large eggs
¼ cup sugar
1½ teaspoons vanilla extract
grated zest of 1 lemon
1½ pounds whole-milk ricotta
2 cups Wheatberries with Fruit and Honey-Orange Dressing
   (page 212)

Preheat oven to 375° F. Generously butter a 9-inch Pyrex pie plate, add the bread crumbs, and coat the bottom and sides, shaking out any excess crumbs.

With an electric mixer, beat the eggs and sugar until they are thick and light. Add the vanilla extract and lemon zest and beat until combined. Add the ricotta and beat on low speed just until mixed. Add the wheatberries and fold in by hand, using a wooden spoon or rubber spatula. Pour and scrape the custard into the pie plate and smooth the top. Bake in the middle of the oven for 40 to 45 minutes, or until the edges are golden brown, the pie is slightly puffed, and a skewer or toothpick inserted in the center comes out clean. Don't overbake. Serve at room temperature.

BLUEBERRY LASSI

❖

Serves 2 (makes about 3 cups)

I prefer to use frozen organic blueberries and a mild-flavored plain yogurt with 1 percent milk fat for this refreshing drink, which is loaded with calcium and high-quality protein.

1½ cups low-fat yogurt
1 cup frozen blueberries
½ cup water
2 teaspoons superfine sugar, or to taste
½ teaspoon orange flower water *or* drops of vanilla

Place all the ingredients in a blender and blend at high speed until the blueberries are pureed and the drink is frothy. The lassi can be stored in the refrigerator for 2 or 3 hours. Serve cold.

SOY FRUIT SMOOTHIE

❖

Serves 2 to 3 (makes 3⅓ to 3½ cups)

2 medium bananas, peeled and cut into chunks
1 cup frozen raspberries or other frozen fruit
2 cups calcium-enriched soy milk
1 tablespoon maple syrup

In a blender, combine all the ingredients at a high speed until the fruits are pureed and the color is uniform.

What's in a Label?

❖

Chicken Rice Soup

Nutrition Facts

Serving Size: 1 cup (238 g)
Servings per container: 2

Amount Per Serving

Calories 90   Calories from Fat 10

% Daily Value*

Total Fat 2g	**3%**
Saturated Fat 0g	**0%**
Cholesterol 10mg	**3%**
Sodium 890mg	**37%**
Total Carbohydrate 13g	**4%**
Dietary Fiber 1g	**4%**
Sugars 1g	
Protein 6g	

Vitamin A 20%   Vitamin C 0%

Calcium 0%   Iron 2%

*Percent Daily Values are based on a 2,000-calorie diet. Your daily values may be higher or lower, depending on your calorie needs.

		Calories	2,000	2,500
Total fat	Less than		65g	80g
Sat. fat	Less than		20g	25g
Cholesterol	Less than		300mg	300mg
Sodium	Less than		2,400mg	2,400mg
Total carbohydrate			300g	375mg
Dietary fiber			25g	30g

Serving size and number of servings per container: The FDA has established specific serving sizes, which reflect the amount a person might typically consume.

Energy, fat, and cholesterol details: It is required that total calories, calories from fat, saturated fat, cholesterol, and sodium be listed in amounts contained per serving. For all except calories and calories from fat, a percent daily value must also be listed, based on a 2,000-calorie-a-day diet.

Carbohydrates, fiber, and sugar: Carbo-hydrate amount must be listed, as well as amount of fiber and sugar that compose those carbohydrates.

Protein: Grams of protein per serving must be listed, but a % daily value is not required here.

Vitamins and minerals: Only vitamins A and C and the minerals calcium and iron must be listed, and % daily values are required rather than actual amounts.

Daily values: If space is available, the % daily values and actual amount for certain nutrients are listed for both 2,000- and 2,500-calorie-a-day diets.

What else is on the label?

Of course there are other elements that make up a food label. An important component is the list of ingredients, which are arranged in descending order by weight. In addition, the name and manufacturer of the product will be listed as well as the common name of the product (i.e., cereal) and descriptive terms such as "cholesterol-free" or "fat-free."

Loopholes in labeling

Though most labels must follow a specific format and provide previously identified important information, some labels may follow the exception to the rule. For instance, if a food container/package has less than forty square inches of surface area, the nutrition label can be abbreviated (but still must contain a minimum of what is included in the above label). While a food container/package with less than twelve square inches of surface area does not need a nutrition label, an address or telephone number must be listed for obtaining that information. Items such as coffee, tea, spices, and foods produced by small businesses or foods prepared and sold within the same business are not required to have a nutrition label, but most will offer such labels voluntarily as they pertain to a particular item. People should also know that restaurants need to provide nutritional information on items they have labeled as low-fat or heart-healthy.

Understanding what the Daily Values (DV) means to you

The FDA developed the DV for the use on food labels to serve as a guide for the needs of the average consumer. Most labels will provide DV based on a 2,000-calorie-a-day diet; however, depending on your individual caloric needs, the percent of calories, fat, nutrients, etc., may be more or less.

If you consume around 2,000 calories a day, then a given serving of a food that provides 10% of the daily value is actually 10% of what you need of that nutrient for the day. However, if you follow a 1,500- or 2,500-calorie-a-day diet, you would want to work toward 75% or 125%, respectively, of each of the items listed because your caloric, fat, and nutrient needs are different.

Other criteria for health claims

In order for a product to make health claims such as "low-fat" or "healthy," certain guidelines must be followed and the product must meet the minimum criteria set forth. Here are a few examples:

High fiber: ≥ 5 g of fiber per serving

Healthy: low in fat, saturated fat, cholesterol, and sodium; $\geq 10\%$ DV for vitamin A, C, iron, calcium, protein and fiber

Good source of: serving provides between 10% and 19% DV for a given nutrient

Fiber Content of Foods

PRODUCT	AMOUNT	FIBER TYPE	DIETARY FIBER (g)
GRAINS			
Bread			
Whole wheat	28 g slice	Insoluble	1.9 g
White	25 g slice	Insoluble	0.6 g
Rye	32 g slice	Insoluble	1.9 g
Cereal			
All bran	½ cup	Insoluble	10 g
Bran flakes	⅔ cup	Insoluble	6 g
Cheerios	1 cup	Soluble	3 g
Corn flakes	1 cup	Insoluble	1.1 g
Raisin bran	1 cup	Insoluble	8.2 g
Oatmeal, old-fashioned	½ cup dry	Soluble	3.7 g
Pasta			
Enriched white	1 cup cooked	Insoluble	2.4 g
Whole wheat	1 cup cooked	Insoluble	6.3 g
Rice			
Brown, long grain	1 cup cooked	Insoluble	3.5 g
White, long grain	1 cup cooked	Insoluble	1.0 g
Bagel			
Oat bran	3.5"	Soluble	2.6 g
Onion, plain, poppy	3.5"	Insoluble	1.6 g

PRODUCT	AMOUNT	FIBER TYPE	DIETARY FIBER (g)
GRAINS			
Pita bread			
White	6.5" diameter	Insoluble	1.3 g
Wheat	6.5" diameter	Insoluble	4.7 g
FRUITS			
Apple	1 med w/ skin	Soluble	3.7 g
Avocado, Florida	1 med, raw	Soluble	16.1 g
Banana	1 med, raw	Soluble	2.7 g
Berries			
Strawberries	1 cup, raw	Soluble	3.4 g
Raspberries	1 cup, raw	Soluble	8.4 g
Blackberries	1 cup, raw	Soluble	7.6 g
Blueberries	1 cup, raw	Soluble	3.9 g
Grapefruit, red or pink	½ med, raw	Soluble	1.4 g
Mango	1 med, raw	Soluble	3.7 g
Pear	1 med, raw	Soluble	4.0 g
VEGETABLES			
Asparagus	6 spears, boiled	Soluble	1.4 g
Broccoli	1 cup, boiled	Soluble	4.6 g
Carrot	1 med, raw	Soluble	2.2 g
Cauliflower	1 cup, boiled	Soluble	3.4 g
Green beans	1 cup, boiled	Soluble	4.0 g
Onions	1 cup, raw, chopped	Soluble	2.8 g
Spinach	1 cup boiled	Soluble	4.4 g
Potato	202 g baked w/ skin	Soluble	4.8 g

PRODUCT	AMOUNT	FIBER TYPE	DIETARY FIBER (g)
LEGUMES			
Beans			
Black	1 cup, boiled	Soluble	15 g
Broad	1 cup, boiled	Soluble	9.2 g
Chickpeas	1 cup, boiled	Soluble	12.5 g
Great northern	1 cup, boiled	Soluble	12.4 g
Kidney	1 cup, boiled	Soluble	13.1 g
Lima	1 cup, boiled	Soluble	13.2 g
Navy	1 cup, boiled	Soluble	11.6 g
Soy	1 cup, boiled	Soluble	10.3 g
Lentils	1 cup, boiled	Soluble	15.6 g
Peas, green	1 cup, frozen, boiled	Soluble	4.4 g
Peas, split	1 cup boiled	Soluble	16.3 g
Edamame	½ cup boiled	Soluble	3.8 g
Soybean products			
Miso	½ cup	Soluble	7.5 g
Natto	½ cup	Soluble	4.8 g
Tempeh	½ cup	—	—
Tofu, firm	½ cup, raw	Soluble	2.9 g

Vitamin and Mineral Index

❖

Nutrient	Purpose/Function	Requirement (DRI/RDA)	Daily Values (DV)	Upper Limit (UL)	Food sources	Comments
Fat-Soluble Vitamins						
Vitamin A	Helps with night vision; may help reduce risk of certain cancers; important in cell growth and function; helps prevent infection	Females: 700 mcg Males: 900 mcg	5,000 IU (1,500 mcg)	3,000 mcg	Vitamin A: animal products such as eggs, milk, fish oil and liver; Beta-carotene: sweet potatoes, carrots, mangos, peppers, and dark green leafy vegetables	Antioxidant; Beta-carotene is converted to vitamin A in the body.
Vitamin D*	Promotes strong teeth and bones by facilitating the absorption of calcium and phosphorus and the mineralization of bone	Males and females Up to age 50: 5 mcg or 200 IU Age 50–70: 10 mcg or 400 IU Past age 70: 15 mcg or 600 IU	400 IU (10 mcg)	50 mcg (or 2,000 IU)	Milk; fortified cereals; small amounts are also found in eggs; sardines; salmon; and margarine	Vitamin D is also produced in the skin via sunlight exposure
Vitamin E* (alpha tocopherol)	May reduce risk of heart disease, cataracts, and cancer; Important for the immune system	Females: 15 mg Males: same	30 IU (9 mg)	1,000 mg	Vegetable oils; nuts; seeds; wheat germ; fish; mangos; papaya; and some green leafy vegetables	Antioxidant; vitamin E found in oils is destroyed during frying
Vitamin K	Assists in blood coagulation; helps produce various other proteins need for blood, bones, and kidneys	Females: 90 mcg Males 120 mcg	80 mcg	— (no upper limit for toxicity established)	Green tea; spinach; broccoli; turnip greens; cauliflower; chickpeas; lentils; and seaweed— dried dulse or rockweed	Some vitamin K is also produced via bacteria in the intestines

Nutrient	Purpose/Function	Requirement (DRI/RDA)	Daily Values (DV)	Upper Limit (UL)	Food sources	Comments
Water-Soluble Vitamins						
Vitamin C* (ascorbic acid)	Assists with the health of: muscles, bones, gums, blood vessels, and capillaries; helps iron absorption; assists in fighting and preventing infections	Females: 75mg Males: 90 mg [+35 mg/day for smokers]	60 mg	2 g	Bell peppers, especially red, orange and yellow; papaya; orange juice; oranges; broccoli; grapefruit; strawberries; melon	Antioxidant; smokers should aim for at least 110–125 mg of vitamin C daily
Biotin*	Energy production; helps the body metabolize protein, fat, and carbohydrates from food	Females: 30 mcg Males: same	300 mcg	— 10 mg**	Eggs; wheat germ; oatmeal; liver	—
Folate* (folic acid or folacin)	DNA and RNA production assisting in new cell formation; helps lower risk of neural tube defects; forms hemoglobin in red blood cells with vitamin B_{12}, may help prevent heart disease and stroke	Females: 400 mcg Males: same	400 mcg	1,000 mcg	Green leafy vegetables; legumes; wheat germ; avocados; oranges; enriched grain products	Especially important for pregnant women and women in the child-bearing years of life as well as for the elderly
Niacin*	Energy production; assists in normal enzyme function and the use of sugars and fatty acids by the body	Females: 14 mg Males: 16 mg	20 mg NE (1 mg NE = 1 mg Niacin or 60 mg tryptophan)	35 mg	Poultry; beef; fish; nuts; legumes; yogurt; and fortified grain products	Only take niacin supple-ments in the prescribed amount
Pantothenic acid*	Energy production; helps the body metabolize protein, fat, and carbohydrates from food	Females: 5 mg Males: same	10 mg	— 10 g**	Fish; poultry; beef; pork; yogurt; eggs; legumes; whole grain cereals; some fruits and vegetables	—

Nutrient	Purpose/Function	Requirement (DRI/RDA)	Daily Values (DV)	Upper Limit (UL)	Food sources	Comments
Pyridoxine* (Vitamin B₆)	Assists in protein insulin, hemoglobin, and antibody production; helps convert amino acids in food into niacin and serotonin	Females Up to age 50: 1.3 mg Past age 50: 1.5 mg Males Up to age 50: 1.3 mg Past age 50: 1.7 mg	2 mg	100 mg	Poultry; pork; nuts; beans; whole grains	—
Cobalamin* (Vitamin B₁₂)	Red blood cell production; assists in the use of sugars and fatty acids by the body; assists in nerve cell maintenance	Females: 2.4 mcg Males: same	6 mcg	100 mcg**	Fish; beef; poultry; dairy products; eggs; some fortified foods	The elderly and vegans are at risk for deficiency; the vitamin is usually destroyed during microwave cooking
Riboflavin* (Vitamin B₂)	Energy production; helps convert amino acids in food into niacin	Females: 1.1 mg Males: 1.3 mg	1.7 mg	— (no upper limit for toxicity established)	Yogurt; milk; liver; eggs; certain grain products	*Myth:* riboflavin deficiency causes hair loss
Thiamin* (Vitamin B₁)	Assists in production of energy from carbohydrates	Females: 1.1 mg Males: 1.2 mg	1.5 mg	— (no upper limit for toxicity established)	Whole grain and enriched grain products; pork; liver	*Myth:* additional thiamin provides extra energy
Minerals						
Calcium*	Builds and strengthens bone; assists in blood clotting, nerve conduction, and muscle contraction	Male and females Up to age 50: 1,000 mg Past age 50: 1,200 mg	1,000 mg	2,500 mg	Milk; yogurt; cheese; kale; spinach; broccoli; bok choy; fish with edible bones; calcium-fortified soy milk and orange juice; tofu made with calcium sulfate	Calcium deficiency can lead to growth retardation and/or osteoporosis

Nutrient	Purpose/Function	Requirement (DRI/RDA)	Daily Values (DV)	Upper Limit (UL)	Food sources	Comments
Magnesium*	Vital component to many body enzymes; important component of muscles and nerve cells as well as bone	Females Up to age 30: 310 mg Past age 30: 320 mg Males Up to age 30: 400 mg Past age 30: 420 mg	400 mg	350 mg from non-food sources (supplements)	Legumes; nuts; whole grains; spinach; parsnips	—
Phosphorus*	Assists in energy production and metabolism; is a component of DNA and RNA as well as a major component of bones and teeth	Females: 700 mg Males: same	1,000 mg	4 g	Dairy products; fish; beef; poultry; legumes; tofu; eggs; most processed foods	*Myth:* Colas and sodas contain excessive amounts of phosphorus, which leads to bone loss (average cola contains 0–45 mg per 12 ounces)
			Trace Elements			
Choline*	Used to make acetylcholine, a neurotransmitter	Females: 425 mg Males: 550 mg	—	3,500 mg	Milk; liver; eggs; peanuts	—
Fluoride*	Assists in hardening tooth enamel and preventing decay; may help reduce risk for osteoporosis	Females: 3 mg Males: 4 mg	—	10 mg	Tea; fish with edible bones	Town water is usually fluoridated; well and bottled waters are generally not
Iodine	Helps to regulate energy utilization	Females: 150 mcg Males: same	150 mcg	— 2 mg**	Salt; saltwater fish such as cod and haddock; very small amount in grain products and some vegetables	Deficiency is uncommon because of the iodization of salt

Nutrient	Purpose/Function	Requirement (DRI/RDA)	Daily Values (DV)	Upper Limit (UL)	Food sources	Comments
Iron	Assists in the delivery of oxygen to the cells of the body; is an essential component of hemoglobin	Females Up to age 50: 18 mg Past age 50: 8 mg Males: 8 mg	18 mg	45 mg	Meats; certain vegetables	Iron is better absorbed from animal sources and when vitamin C is also consumed
Selenium*	Helps with cell growth; works with vitamin E to help prevent cancer, heart disease, and other diseases	Females: 55 mcg Males: same	70 mcg	400 mcg	Seafood; poultry; whole-grain products; eggs	Works as an antioxidant with vitamin E
Manganese	Component of several enzymes	Females: 1.8 mg Males: 2.3 mg	2 mg	11 mg	Whole-grain foods; pineapple; lentils; strawberries; kale	—
Molybdenum	Component of several enzymes; assists in using iron stored in the body to produce hemoglobin to make red blood cells	45 mcg	75 mcg	2,000 mcg	Milk; legumes; liver	—
Chromium	Assists in blood sugar utilization along with insulin	Females Up to age 50: 25 mcg Past age 50: Males: 35 mcg	120 mcg	—	Meat; eggs; whole-grain foods; peas; cheese; eggs	Deficiency can mirror diabetes
Copper	Helps in the production of energy and hemoglobin; is an important component of several enzymes	900 mcg	2 mg	10,000 mcg	Liver; fish; nuts; legumes; seeds	—

Nutrient	Purpose/Function	Requirement (DRI/RDA)	Daily Values (DV)	Upper Limit (UL)	Food sources	Comments
Zinc	Essential for cell and tissue growth and repair; component of many enzymes; helps the body metabolize protein, fat, and carbohydrates from food; important for the immune system	Females: 8 mg Males: 11 mg	15 mg	40 mg	Beef; seafood; tofu; legumes; nuts; seeds; milk; eggs	Adequate zinc is important to prevent birth defects and promote proper growth during childhood
Electrolytes						
Sodium	Helps with fluid and blood pressure regulation, nerve signal transmission, and muscle relaxation	500 mg	2,400 mg	2,400 mg	Processed foods; salt; cheese; bread; milk	¼ teaspoon of salt provides 500 mg of sodium
Potassium	Assists in muscle contraction, normal blood pressure maintenance, nerve signal transmission, and fluid and mineral balance regulation		3,500 mg	— 18 g**	Bananas; milk; fish; legumes; potatoes; squash; apricots; oranges; melon	While there is no RDA for potassium, 2,000–3,500 mg daily is recommended; less processed foods usually have more potassium
Chloride	Aids in digestion and absorption of nutrients; helps in regulation and the transmission of nerve signals	750 mg	3,400 mg	— (RDA book does not recommend any upper limit at all!)	Salt; salty foods	¼ teaspoon of salt provides 750 fluid mg of chloride

*Most up-to-date DRI values.
**While an official upper limit has not been established, this is the amount at which toxicity is thought to occur.

VITAMINS AND MINERALS

Vitamins are organic chemical nutrients found in food. They are essential in small amounts for the body to function properly.

Fat-soluble vitamins (A, D, E, and K) are stored until they are needed in the body's fatty tissues and in the liver. Because they are stored for longer periods than water-soluble vitamins, it is not necessary to consume them every day.

Water-soluble vitamins (C and the B vitamins) move freely throughout the bloodstream. Because the excess is excreted via the kidneys, water-soluble vitamins must be consumed more regularly.

Minerals are inorganic chemical nutrients that are found in the body in amounts of at least 5 grams.

Trace elements are minerals that are found in the body in amounts of less than 5 grams.

Electrolytes are salts and other minerals that dissolve in water and help regulate fluid balance and acid base in the body.

RDAs—Recommended Daily Allowances

Since 1941, the RDAs, prepared by the Food and Nutrition Board of the National Academy of Sciences, have been the benchmark of recommendations for various nutrient intakes. The traditional role of the RDA is described by its definition adopted more than twenty years ago: "The levels of intake of essential nutrients that, on the basis of scientific knowledge, are judged by the Food and Nutrition Board to be adequate to meet the known nutrient needs of practically all healthy persons." Up until a few years ago they were recognized in the food and health fields as the accepted source on nutrient allowances. The RDAs, which have been revised over the years to reflect current research, are now being replaced by Dietary Reference Intakes (DRIs), but until all the DRI values have been established, RDAs will continue to be included in the standards referred to on the Nutrition Facts labels that appear on all packaged foods.

DRIs—Dietary Reference Intakes

Since the last publication of the RDAs in 1989, there has been increasing awareness of the impact of nutrition on chronic disease. Because of the new research findings and a growing public focus on nutrition and health, the expert panel within the Food and Nutrition Board at the National Academy of Sciences has reviewed and expanded its approach, and the result is the new Dietary Reference Intakes (DRIs). The DRIs are being developed jointly by U.S. and Canadian scientists and will greatly extend the scope and use of the previous nutrient guidelines. There have been four sets of DRIs released to date. Over the next few years, all of the nutrient guidelines will be revised, and will include new recommendations for fiber and some phytochemicals.

UL—Upper Limit

Also known as the Tolerable Upper Intake Limits, these are the values assigned to suggest the maximum safe level of intake of a nutrient, one that will not put people at risk for adverse effects. Only nutrients that have a DRI have a designated UL.

Daily Value or DV

Daily values were established specifically for food label use to reflect the dietary recommendations for nutrients and dietary components that have important relationships with health. The percent daily value column within a food label provides an estimate of how individual foods contribute to the total diet. In general, daily values are based on a 2,000-calorie diet, though they can be adjusted to accommodate higher or lower caloric diets.

Resources

❖

The resources here will lead you to more information about particular issues. This is a list of organizations, names and addresses, books, and websites. Please bear in mind that websites come and go. The sites listed here were accessible when I compiled this section. If any one of them is inoperative at a later date, use a reliable search engine to locate the source at its new site. I also encourage you to go to my website, *www.StrongWomen.com*.

FOOD GUIDE PYRAMID AND DIETARY GUIDELINES

The following website contains information regarding the Food Guide Pyramid. If you scroll to the bottom of the page, you will find a number of the alternative FGPs.

www.nal.usda.gov/fnic/Fpyr/pyramid.html

Single copies of *Nutrition and Your Health: Dietary Guidelines for Americans, Fifth Edition (2000)* are available for $4.75 each from the Consumer Information Center (Item 147G). Order online or call 888-878-3256 (M–F, 9:00 am to 8:00 pm Eastern time).

health.gov/dietaryguidelines

Or view the guidelines online through Adobe Acrobat at:

health.gov/dietaryguidelines/dga2000/DIETGD.PDF

www.usda.gov/cnpp/Pubs/DG2000/How2Order.html (provides additional information for ordering copies of the 2000 guidelines)

Oldways is an organization interested in raising public awareness of Mediterranean and vegetarian diets, among other dietary options, and it is an originator of a number of alternative food guide pyramids.

Oldways Preservation & Exchange Trust

266 Beacon Street, Boston, MA 02116

Tel: 617-421-5500; fax: 617-421-5511

www.oldways@oldwayspt.org

Experts at Tufts University review and rank websites that contain nutrition information through a Tufts-sponsored website.

navigator.tufts.edu

GENERAL NUTRITION RESOURCES

Three books with reliable current information:

Understanding Nutrition, Eighth Edition, Eleanor Noss Whitney and Sharon Rady Rolfes. Belmont, CA: Wadsworth, 1999.

The American Dietetic Association's Complete Food & Nutrition Guide, Roberta Larson Duyff. Minneapolis: Chronimed Publishing, 1996, 1998.

Lifestyle Nutrition, edited by James M. Rippe and Johanna T. Dwyer. Boston: Blackwell Scientific, 2000.

Four government websites:

Team Nutrition

www.usda.gov/fcs/team.htm

This government site is a total resource for support groups, treatment options, and other necessary information.

National Cancer Institute

www.nci.nih.gov/

National Institutes of Health
www.nih.gov/

U.S. Department of Agriculture
Food and Nutrition Information Center
www.nal.usda.gov/fnic/

Everything from finding a dietitian to information on policy and scientific research can be accessed on this excellent site:

American Dietetic Association
www.eatright.org/index.html

WATER RESOURCES

Environmental Protection Agency hotline: 800-426-4791
EPA Office of Water
www.epa.org.ow

National Sanitation Foundation
www.nsf.org

Water Quality Association
www.wqa.org

KEGEL EXERCISES

The Mayo Clinic
www.mayohealth.org/mayo/9801/htm/incontirv.htm

The Iowa Women's Health
obgyn.uihc.uiowa.edu/Patinfo/urogyn/kegel.htm

THE NURSES' HEALTH STUDY

The home page of the Nurses' Health Study at Brigham and Women's Hospital in Boston.
www.channing.harvard.edu/nhs/

OSTEOPOROSIS

The National Osteoporosis Foundation (NOF)
1232 22nd Street, N.W.
Washington, DC 20037-1292
Tel: 800-223-9944 or 202-223-2226
www.nof.org

Strong Women, Strong Bones, Miriam E. Nelson, Ph.D., with Sarah Wernick, Ph.D. New York: Putnam, 2000.

SOY

There are countless organizations and websites with information about soy foods. Here are a few of them. (For others, use a search engine such as *www.google.com.*)

Indiana Soybean Council
www.soyfoods.com

Federal Department of Agriculture (FDA)
www.fda.gov/fdac/features/2000/300_soy.html

U.S. Soyfoods Directory
www.soyfoods.com

SODIUM

This is the FDA website on sodium:
www.fda.gov/fdac/foodlabel/sodium.html

COOKING EQUIPMENT

This is a resource for whetstones to sharpen knives:
DMT—Diamond Machining Technology, Inc.
85 Hayes Memorial Drive
Marlborough, MA 01752-1892
www.DMTSharp.com

A handsome and very readable reference to cooking equipment is:
The New Cooks' Catalogue, edited by Burt Wolfe, Emily Aronson, and
Florence Fabricant. New York: Knopf, 2000.

ORGANIC AND WHOLE FOODS/
GENETICALLY ENGINEERED OR MODIFIED FOODS

Organizations concerned with organic foods are very often equally con-
cerned with and about genetically engineered foods.
BioDemocracy and Organic Consumers Association
6101 Cliff Estate Road
Little Marais, MN 55614
E-mail: biodemocracy@mail.eworld3.net
Staff Activist or Media Inquiries: 218-226-4164; fax: 218-226-4157
www.purefood.org

Environmental Working Group
1716 Connecticut Ave. NW
Washington, DC 20009
e-mail: *info@ewg.org* Website: *www.foodnews.org*

This website has a shopping list for non-GE foods and a source for GE/GM food news updates.
Greenpeace
True Food Now
Tel: 800-219-9260
www.truefoodnow.org

COOKBOOKS

These three books are a useful addition to any cookbook library.

An excellent general cookbook that actually lives up to the promise of its title:

How to Cook Everything: Simple Recipes for Great Food, Mark Bittman. New York: Macmillan, 1998.

Madhur Jaffrey's World Vegetarian. New York: Clarkson Potter, 1999.

This Can't Be Tofu! Deborah Madison. New York: Broadway Books, 2000.

ORGANIC AND NONORGANIC FOOD

The best way to find sources for organic foods is to bring a pad and pencil to take down names, addresses, and websites when you visit a health-food store.

Packagers of a wide range of organic foods:
Eden Foods
Clinton, MI 49236
Tel: 888-441-EDEN (3336) or 888-424-EDEN (3336)
www.eden-foods.com

Producers and packagers of organic rices:

Lundberg Family Farms

5370 Church St.

Box 369

Richvale, CA 95974-0369

Tel: 530-882-4451; fax: 530-882-4500

www.lundberg.com/home.html

Two mills that stone-grind grits, one of the foods I love most:

Falls Mills

134 Falls Mill Rd.

Belvidere, TN 37306

Tel: 931-469-7161

www.fallsmill.com

Nora Mill Granary

7107 South Main Street

Helen, GA 30545

Tel: 800-927-2375

www.noramill.com

This organic food conglomerate owns a number of smaller companies, such as Arrowhead Mills, Health Valley Foods, and Hain Pure Foods.

Hain Food Group

1 Dalewood Way

San Francisco, CA 94127-1605

Tel: 415-587-7198; fax: 415-587-7199

www.thehainfoodgroup.com

An extraordinary source for spices and condiments, from curry leaves to Persian saffron, as well as more than 30 rices and over 45 varieties of dried beans. Worth a detour if you visit New York.

Kalustyan's
123 Lexington Ave.
New York, NY 10016
Tel: 212-685-3451; fax: 212-683-8458
Home page: *www.kalustyans.com*
Spices: *www.forspice.com*
Rice and dried beans: *www.riceandbeans.com*

Deservedly famous for their vast array of spices:
Penzey's Spices
P.O. Box 933
Muskego, WI 53150
Tel: 800-741-7787; fax: 262-679-7878
www.penzeys.com

Heirloom beans, grains, and other products:
Indian Harvest of Bemidji, Minn.
800-346-7032
www.indianharvest.com

Dried heirloom beans, sold by harvest date (the more recent the date, the
tenderer and more flavorful the bean):
Phipps Country Store & Farm
P.O. Box 349
Pescadero, CA 94060
Tel: (local) 415-879-0787; (toll-free) 800-279-0889 (mail order only)

Premium fresh and dried wild mushrooms, truffles, and other divinely delicious foods. Call or e-mail for brochure.
Urbani USA
29-24 40th Ave.
Long Island City, NY 11101
Tel: 800-281-2330
e-mail: *urbaniusa@aol.com*
www.urbani.com

Index

ABOUT THE AUTHORS

Miriam Nelson, Ph.D., author of the international bestsellers *Strong Women Stay Young, Strong Women Stay Slim,* and *Strong Women, Strong Bones,* is associate professor of nutrition at the School of Nutrition Science and Policy and director of the Center for Physical Fitness at Tufts University. Dr. Nelson holds the title of fellow of the American College of Sports Medicine, an honor reserved for those who have demonstrated superior leadership and research in the field of exercise. Her original research papers on nutrition and exercise have been published in distinguished peer-reviewed journals, including the *Journal of the American Medical Association.* In 1994 she was named a Brookdale National Fellow; this prestigious recognition is given annually to only five or six young scholars in the field of aging. She was a Bunting Fellow at Radcliffe College in 1997–1998. In 2000, her *Strong Women, Strong Bones* received the Books for a Better Life Award for best wellness book from the Multiple Sclerosis Society. Dr. Nelson has been featured on many television and radio programs, including the *Today* show, *Good Morning America,* and *Fresh Air,* and on CNN. The founder of *www.StrongWomen.com,* she lives in Concord, Massachusetts, with her husband and three children.

Judy Knipe is the author of *Sensational Soups* and a coauthor of the *Christmas Cookie Book.* She lives in New York City.